T0295393

Pressure Injuries and Chronic Wounds

Editor

JEFFREY M. LEVINE

CLINICS IN GERIATRIC MEDICINE

www.geriatric.theclinics.com

Consulting Editor
G. MICHAEL HARPER

August 2024 • Volume 40 • Number 3

ELSEVIER

1600 John F. Kennedy Boulevard • Suite 1800 • Philadelphia, Pennsylvania, 19103-2899

http://www.theclinics.com

CLINICS IN GERIATRIC MEDICINE Volume 40, Number 3
August 2024 ISSN 0749–0690, ISBN-13: 978-0-443-24650-0

Editor: Taylor Hayes
Developmental Editor: Anita Chamoli

Clinics in Geriatric Medicine (ISSN 0749-0690) is published quarterly by Elsevier Inc., 360 Park Avenue South, New York, NY 10010-1710. Months of issue are February, May, August, and November. Business and Editorial Offices: 1600 John F. Kennedy Blvd., Suite 1800, Philadelphia, PA 191023-2899. Periodicals postage paid at New York, NY, and additional mailing offices. Subscription prices are $321.00 per year (US individuals), $100.00 per year (US & Canadian student/resident), $340.00 per year (Canadian individuals), $457.00 per year (international individuals), and $195.00 per year (international student/resident). For institutional access pricing please contact Customer Service via the contact information below. Foreign air speed delivery is included in all *Clinics* subscription prices. All prices are subject to change without notice. POSTMASTER: Send address changes to *Clinics in Geriatric Medicine,* Elsevier Health Sciences Division, Subscription Customer Service, 3251 Riverport Lane, Maryland Heights, MO 63043. **Telephone: 1-800-654-2452 (U.S. and Canada); 314-447-8871 (outside U.S. and Canada). Fax: 314-447-8029. E-mail:** journalscustomerservice-usa@elsevier.com **(for print support) or** journalsonlinesupport-usa@elsevier.com **(for online support).**

Reprints. For copies of 100 or more, of articles in this publication, please contact the Commercial Reprints Department, Elsevier Inc., 360 Park Avenue South, New York, New York 10010-1710. Tel.: 212-633-3874; Fax: 212-633-3820, E-mail: reprints@elsevier.com.

Clinics in Geriatric Medicine is covered in *MEDLINE/PubMed (Index Medicus), EMBASE/Excerpta Medica, Current Contents/Clinical Medicine (CC/CM), and the Cumulative Index to Nursing & Allied Health Literature.*

Contributors

CONSULTING EDITOR

G. MICHAEL HARPER, MD
Professor of Medicine, Geriatrics Department of Medicine, University of California, San Francisco, San Francisco, California, USA

EDITOR

JEFFREY M. LEVINE, MD, AGSF, CMD, CWS-P
Clinical Professor of Geriatric Medicine and Palliative Care, Department of Geriatrics, Icahn School of Medicine at Mount Sinai, New York, New York, USA

AUTHORS

MARNIE ABESHOUSE, MD
Senior Surgical Resident, Department of Surgery, Icahn School of Medicine at Mount Sinai, New York, New York, USA

WAHILA ALAM, MD, CMS
Assistant Professor, Department of Geriatrics, University of Connecticut, Farmington, Connecticut, USA

SCOTT MATTHEW BOLHACK, MD, MBA, CMD, CWSP, PCWC, FACP
Chief Medical Officer, TLC HealthCare Wound Consultants, Tucson, Arizona, USA

BARBARA DELMORE, PhD, RN, CWCN, MAPWCA, IIWCC-NYU, FAAN
Senior Nurse Scientist, Department of Nursing, Center for Innovations in the Advancement of Care, NYU Langone Health; Clinical Assistant Professor, Hansjörg Wyss, Department of Plastic Surgery, NYU Grossman School of Medicine, New York, New York, USA

CORNELIUS MICHAEL DONOHUE, DPM, ACFAS
President, World Walk Foundation, Ardmore, Pennsylvania, USA

ALLEGRA L. FIERRO, MD
Vascular and Wound Repair Clinical Research Fellow, Department of Surgery, Icahn School of Medicine at Mount Sinai, New York, New York, USA

AIMEE D. GARCIA, MD, CWS, MAPWCA
Associate Professor, Department of Medicine, Baylor College of Medicine; Medical Director, Wound Clinic and Consult Service, Michael E. DeBakey VA Medical Center, Houston, Texas, USA

LISA J. GOULD, MD, PhD
Clinical Associate Professor, The Warren Alpert Medical School of Brown University, Providence, Rhode Island, USA; Plastic Surgeon, Department of Surgery, South Shore Health, Weymouth, Massachusetts, USA

SARWAT JABEEN, MD
Faculty physician, Michael E. DeBakey Department of Veterans Affairs, Houston, Texas, USA; Teaching Faculty, Department of Family Medicine, Memorial Hermann Family Medicine Residency Program, Sugar Land

TOMER LAGZIEL, MD
Surgical Intern, Department of Surgery, Icahn School of Medicine at Mount Sinai, New York, New York, USA

JOHN C. LANTIS II, MD
Chief and Professor, Department of Surgery, Icahn School of Medicine at Mount Sinai, Mount Sinai West, New York, New York, USA

JEFFREY M. LEVINE, MD, AGSF, CMD, CWS-P
Clinical Professor of Geriatric Medicine and Palliative Care, Department of Geriatrics, Icahn School of Medicine at Mount Sinai, New York, New York, USA

MARY LITCHFORD, PhD, RDN
President, Case Software, Greensboro, North Carolina, USA

NANCY MUNOZ, DCN, MHA, RDN, FAND
UMass Amherst Instructor, Rosalind Franklin University of Medicine and Science, Chicago, Illinois, USA; Adjunct Assistant Professor, Chief Nutrition and Food Service, VA Southern Nevada Healthcare System, Las Vegas, Nevada, USA

NATALIE E. NIERENBERG, MD, MPH
Director, Wound Care, Department of Infectious Diseases, Tufts Medical Center, Boston, Massachusetts, USA

ARTHUR STONE, DPM
President, MedNexus, Inc., Greenville, South Carolina, USA

ELIZABETH FOY WHITE CHU, MD, CWSP, AGSF
Associate Professor, Department of Medicine, Oregon Health and Sciences University, Medical Director, Wound Healing Service, Portland VA Health Care System, Portland, Oregon, USA

KEVIN WOO, PhD, RN, NSWOC, WOCC(C)
Professor, Faculty of Health Sciences, Queen's University, Kingston, Ontario, Canada

Contents

Care for the older patient living with a chronic wound comes with challenges not seen in younger patients. The aging skin, impacted by the environment and intrinsic physiologic changes, makes it susceptible to injury and poor healing. Likewise, older adults' goals with regards to wound healing may vary depending on their functional abilities and quality of life. The clinician must pay attention to these nuances and collaborate with the older patient in developing a treatment plan. Careful systematic description, documentation, and communication with the patient/caregiver aids the clinician in tracking the treatment goals and potentially reducing medical liability risk.

Wound healing is a highly complex natural process, and its failure results in chronic wounds. The causes of delayed wound healing include patient-related and local wound factors. The main local impediments to delayed healing are the presence of nonviable tissue, excessive inflammation, infection, and moisture imbalance. For wounds that can be healed with adequate blood supply, a stepwise approach to identify and treat these barriers is termed wound bed preparation. Currently, a combination of patient-related and local factors, including wound debridement, specialty dressings, and advanced technologies, is available and successfully used to facilitate the healing process.

Pressure injuries are a common chronic wound in the older adult. Care of pressure injuries is an interprofessional effort and involves physicians, nurses, registered dieticians, rehabilitation therapists, and surgical subspecialties. Numerous treatment modalities exist but have varying evidence to substantiate their efficacy. All primary and other care providers, particularly geriatricians, need to be aware of current evidence-based prevention and treatment standards. When healing is not expected, palliative care should be considered to avoid futile procedures and preserve dignity and quality of life.

The physical, emotional, and financial toll of acute and chronic nonhealing wounds on older adults and their caregivers is immense. Surgical treatment of wounds in older adults can facilitate healing but must consider the medical complexity of the patient, the patient's desires for treatment and the likelihood of healing. Innovative approaches and devices can promote rapid healing. By using a team approach, from preoperative planning to postoperative care, with a focus on the needs and desires of the patient, successful outcomes with improved patient satisfaction are possible even in medically complex patients.

The treatment, maintenance, and suppression of infection in chronic wounds remain a challenge to all practitioners. From an infectious disease standpoint, knowing when a chronic wound has progressed from colonized to infected, when to use systemic antimicrobial therapy and when and how to culture such wounds can be daunting. With few standardized clinical guidelines for infections in chronic wounds, caring for them is an art form. However, there have been notable advances in the diagnosis, treatment, and management of infected wounds. This article will discuss the pathophysiology of infection in older adults, including specific infections such as cutaneous candidiasis, necrotizing soft tissue infection, osteomyelitis, and infections involving hardware.

Malnutrition is a collective term that includes both undernutrition and malnutrition. Malnutrition presents with and without inflammation, is reported in underweight, normal weight, and overweight individuals, and is associated with undesirable alterations in body composition, and diminished functional status. Older adults commonly experience dwindling nutritional status as evidenced by insidious weight loss, insufficient dietary intake, loss of muscle mass, quality, and strength, declining functional status, and other physical and emotional decline indicators. Sustained pressure, acute trauma, malnutrition, and inflammatory-driven chronic conditions increase the risk for skin integrity issues.

Chronic wound–related pain is a complex biopsychosocial experience that is experienced spontaneously at rest and exacerbated during activities. Tissue debridement, trauma at dressing change, increased bioburden or infection, exposure of periwound skin to moisture, and related treatment can modulate chronic wound–related pain. Clinicians should consider multimodal and multidisciplinary management approach that take into account the biology, emotions, cognitive thinking, social environment, and other personal determinants of pain. Unresolved pain can have a significant impact on wound healing, patients' adherence to treatment, and individual's quality of life.

CLINICS IN GERIATRIC MEDICINE

THE CLINICS ARE AVAILABLE ONLINE!
Access your subscription at:
www.theclinics.com

Foreword

Healing the Miseducation About Pressure Injuries and Chronic Wounds

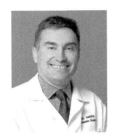

G. Michael Harper, MD
Consulting Editor

My great aunt was a career US Air Force nurse who served during World War II. I was in medical school when I encountered my first patient with a pressure injury, and I have a vivid memory of her reaction when I told her about it. She was quite literally shocked, sharing that it would have been scandalous if an injured airman or soldier developed a pressure injury. She said it would have been considered a failure of care. Because most pressure injuries today occur in older adults who often are frail, have multiple chronic conditions and limited mobility, that viewpoint has evolved, and I while I don't believe most experts would say that all pressure injuries are unavoidable, it's fair to say that with appropriate care, many are preventable.

This issue's guest editor, Dr. Jeffrey Levine, rightfully points out that little time is devoted to pressure injuries and chronic wounds in medical education, and in many institutions the clinical expertise for chronic wound care resides in nursing. For physicians to be effective partners with our nursing colleagues and all members of the interprofessional team in the care of chronic wounds, we must have a basic understanding their pathophysiology and causes, how to prevent and treat them, and when to seek expert consultation.

This issue of *Clinics in Geriatric Medicine* is a comprehensive review of pressure injuries and other chronic wounds, including arterial and venous leg ulcers and diabetic foot ulcers. You will learn about the infectious and surgical aspects of chronic wounds and wound care and the role nutrition plays. There are articles that address the importance of wound bed preparation, treatment approaches, and pain assessment. While it may not be scandalous for an acutely ill, older adult to develop a pressure injury as it may have once been for a World War II airman or soldier, by educating ourselves on the

Clin Geriatr Med 40 (2024) ix–x
https://doi.org/10.1016/j.cger.2024.04.001
0749-0690/24/Published by Elsevier Inc.

fundamentals of pressure injuries and chronic wounds, we can do a better job of preventing and alleviating the suffering associated with them.

G. Michael Harper, MD
Geriatrics Department of Medicine
University of California, San Francisco
4150 Clement Street, Rm 310B
San Francisco, CA 94121, USA

E-mail address:
Michael.harper@ucsf.edu

Preface

Pressure Injuries and Chronic Wounds

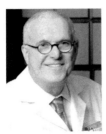

Jeffrey M. Levine, MD, AGSF, CMD, CWS-P
Editor

Pressure injuries (also referred to as bedsores, decubitus ulcers, pressure sores, or pressure ulcers) were designated a geriatric syndrome in the late twentieth century, as they satisfy the criteria of being highly prevalent, multifactorial, and associated with substantial morbidity and poor outcomes.[1,2] In the ensuing decades the topic of pressure injuries lagged as research and knowledge of other geriatric syndromes, such as delirium, dementia, and falls, moved forward.[3] In the face of increased prevalence of chronic diseases, other wounds, such as diabetic foot ulcers, arterial and venous ulcers, and postsurgical and malignant wounds, have increased with substantial overlap of treatments and management decisions. Today, wound care receives little attention in medical training, and many primary care providers—including geriatricians—are often poorly equipped to care for these entities that result in an array of adverse outcomes. Because of their common occurrence in persons of advanced age, geriatricians are in an ideal position to assume the lead in caring for pressure injuries and chronic wounds, and thus the need for this issue.

Wound care is a truly interdisciplinary specialty that requires a team approach and engagement of the patient and their support system. Treatment involves a variety of medical and surgical subspecialists, nutritionists, nurses, and rehabilitation personnel, including occupational therapy, physical therapy, and speech therapy. The spectrum of knowledge required for decision making includes wound assessment, differential diagnosis, pathophysiology of wound healing, palliative care, wound bed preparation, and the formulary of wound care products and technologies. The clinician must be aware of the scope of knowledge and expertise of subspecialties, including

Clin Geriatr Med 40 (2024) xi–xiii
https://doi.org/10.1016/j.cger.2023.12.007
0749-0690/24/© 2023 Published by Elsevier Inc.

geriatric.theclinics.com

dermatology, general surgery, plastic surgery, vascular surgery, and podiatry, to collaborate effectively for the most optimum patient outcome.

Wound care involves addressing complex health needs that render assessment and decision making challenging. These include examining patients who are immobile and in pain, shepherding patients through transitions between care settings, rendering decisions based on the values and goals of patients and families, educating patients and families on treatment choices that may include aggressive and sometimes futile procedures, and coordinating care between multiple providers. A patient-centered approach incorporates the 4Ms—what Matters, Medication, Mind, and Mobility, which organizes complex care for older people based on what is important to them.[4]

Successful wound care requires the clinician be familiar with processes, regulations, and limitations imposed by components of the health care continuum, including outpatient, assisted living, skilled nursing and postacute long-term care, long-term acute care hospitals, and acute care hospitals. The practice of person-centered care requires the clinician be aware of the cultural and economic aspects of wound care as well as associated psychiatric and psychosocial issues.

A chronic wound in an older adult requires the clinical to be aware of the prompt assessment and recognition, including entry into the practitioner's problem list. Critical decisions include when to call consultants, which consultants to call, whether to harness advanced wound-healing technologies and perform aggressive procedures, and realistic patient and family education must be part of the process. To accomplish informed assessment and decision making, the clinician must be knowledgeable regarding the pathophysiologic processes of wound healing and the impact of concomitant comorbidities. The breadth of required knowledge and skill combined with poor representation in medical training can lead the practitioner to sidestep critical issues or delegate decision making to other providers who may be unequipped to handle the true scope and complexity of critical wound-related issues.

For this issue of *Clinics in Geriatric Medicine*, I invited leaders in the field to share their knowledge and expertise with the goal of educating clinicians on the basics of wound care. It is both an honor and a privilege to have the opportunity to bring together information that will improve care of vulnerable adults in an area where it is most needed.

Jeffrey M. Levine, MD, AGSF, CMD, CWS-P
Department of Geriatrics
Icahn School of Medicine at Mount Sinai
1 Gustave L. Levy Pl
New York, NY 10029, USA

E-mail address:
jlevinemd@shcny.com

REFERENCES

1. Bergstrom N, Braden B. A prospective study of pressure sore risk among institutionalized elderly. J Am Geriatr Soc 1992;40:747–58. https://doi.org/10.1111/j.1532-5415.1992.tb01845.x.

2. Inouye SK, Studenski S, Tinetti ME, et al. Geriatric syndromes: clinical, research, and policy implications of a core geriatric concept. J Am Geriatr Soc 2007;55(5):780–91. https://doi.org/10.1111/j.1532-5415.2007.01156.x. PMID: 17493201; PMCID: PMC2409147.

3. Levine JM, Samuels E, Le S, Spinner R. Pressure injuries and wound care: A lost geriatric syndrome. J Am Geriatr Soc. 2024 May 13. https://doi.org/10.1111/jgs. 18969. [Epub ahead of print]. PMID: 38738801.
4. Mate K, Fulmer T, Pelton L, et al. Evidence for the 4Ms: interactions and outcomes across the care continuum. J Aging Health 2021;33(7–8):469–81. https://doi.org/ 10.1177/0898264321991658. PMID: 33555233; PMCID: PMC8236661.

The Challenge of Chronic Wounds in Older Adults

Aimee D. Garcia, MD, CWS, MAPWCA[a,b,*],
Elizabeth Foy White Chu, MD, CWSP, AGSF[c]

KEYWORDS

• Wound healing • Aged • Skin • Chronic wounds

KEY POINTS

- Aging skin creates unique challenges in wound healing in the older adult.
- Cellular and physiologic changes in the healing cascade are impacted by the aging process.
- Be consistent and systematic in wound documentation.
- Communication and documentation are the cornerstones for decreasing the risk of litigation in chronic wound management.

INTRODUCTION

Wound healing encompasses an intricate spectrum of care. Most chronic wounds found in older individuals are a result of complex medical and health-related social needs that predispose this population to skin breakdown. Geriatric medicine is especially poised to co-manage these patients with rehabilitative, surgical, and other medical specialty colleagues. Geriatric medicine training focuses not only on the disease process itself, but also on how older adults navigate health-related social issues such as food security, transportation, social isolation, and housing. Geriatricians constantly coordinate their patients' transition through systems of care at home, in the hospital, and in post-acute rehabilitation facilities. As such, geriatricians take a holistic approach to the management of chronic wounds and focus on them in the context of a geriatric syndrome.

To structure the assessment and management of chronic wounds as a geriatric syndrome, the authors outline them in the context of the Age Friendly model of the 4 M's-

[a] Department of Medicine, Baylor College of Medicine; [b] Wound Clinic and Consult Service, Michael E. DeBakey VA Medical Center, 2002 Holcombe Boulevard, Houston, TX 77030, USA; [c] Department of Geriatrics, Oregon Health & Science University, Portland VA Health Care System, 3710 SW, US Veterans Hospital Road, Portland, OR 97239, USA
* Corresponding author. Wound Clinic and Consult Service, Michael E. DeBakey VA Medical Center, 2002 Holcombe Boulevard, Houston, TX 77030.
E-mail address: aimeeg@bcm.edu

Clin Geriatr Med 40 (2024) 367–373
https://doi.org/10.1016/j.cger.2023.12.008
0749-0690/24/© 2024 Elsevier Inc. All rights reserved.

geriatric.theclinics.com

What Matters Most, Medication, Mentation, and Mobility.[1] Guidelines for the major types of wounds address the generic aspects of prevention and treatment but fail to consider the additional aspects of management more likely to be seen in older adults. The "Age Friendly Health System" is a growing movement and the 4 M's interconnect to support a health care system that is markedly more patient centered.[1] Evidence regarding each individual "M" has suggested there are better health outcomes as well.[2]

To slow down the patient encounter and get to the root of what matters most to the patient, the clinician should consider patient-centered questions that are largely impacted by living with a chronic wound. For those patients labeled as "non-compliant," these questions may illuminate the true barriers to the patient's healing process. **Table 1** illustrates some examples of questions to use for these patients.

AGING SKIN

Although aging affects all organ systems, the most visible signs occur in the skin. Noticeable changes include wrinkling of the skin, thinning of the epidermal layer, loss of subcutaneous fat, and thinning of the hair.[3] Both intrinsic and extrinsic factors impact these changes. Extrinsic changes are a result of environmental influences such as ultraviolet (UV) exposure, exposure to tobacco smoke, and pollution in the air. Intrinsic changes are the result of the aging process and include decreased dermal-epidermal turnover, flattening of the rete ridges, decrease in dermal mast cells, decrease in fibroblasts, and decreased collagen production.[4]

As a physical barrier, the skin provides protection against the external environment, helps to regulate temperature, and prevents fluid losses.[5] Physiologic changes occur in all levels of the skin with aging. In the epidermis, there is flattening of the dermal-epidermal junction. There is also an overall decrease in Langerhan's cells. Keratinocytes, a key component in cell signaling during the healing of a wound, take 50% longer to migrate from the basal membrane to the epithelial layer in older individuals.[6] In the dermal layer, where most wound healing cell lines are found, there are many cellular and physiologic changes. There is an overall decrease in dermal blood flow and microcirculation, which translates to a decreased ability to adapt to temperature changes and respond to injury. The combination of physical and cellular changes combined with underlying medical conditions impacts the integrity of the skin and affect overall wound healing.

CHRONIC WOUNDS

Despite the term "chronic wound," this term is not universally well defined. Some researchers define it as a wound that fails to close in an orderly and timely manner. But timely can be quite subjective, with some studies listing 4 weeks, others 6 or more.[7] This ambiguity has led to difficulties with epidemiologic studies and a lack of focus on prevalence or incidence. Despite this challenge, many studies indicate that chronic wounds increase in prevalence with age regardless of etiology.[8] Latest Medicare expenditures reveal that 16.4% of Medicare beneficiaries have been affected by a chronic wound.[9]

At a cellular level, wound healing reveals a complex process of overlapping phases—inflammation, proliferation, angiogenesis, epidermal restoration, and wound maturation or contraction.[10] These processes are by no means linear and can circle back and forth, with feedback mechanisms in each phase. In chronic wounds, cells act more senescent and do not progress as expected.[7] The literature often discusses the following cells and concepts around wound healing at the microscopic level.

Table 1
"What matters most" example questions

Common Questions for all Wounds	Chronic Wound Syndrome	Specific Questions per Syndrome Type
What part of your wound care is a burden to you?	Pressure injuries	How important is it to you to be able to sit for a few hours, knowing that this may prevent or worsen healing?
What worries you most about the wound? [If they state "I don't know", you can ask about infection, healing, pain]	Venous leg ulcers	How does wearing compression affect your life?
What activities do you want to do that you think the wound prevents you from doing?		How does the drainage affect your day to day life?
What is the one thing about your wound you most want to focus on so that you can do [fill in desired activity] more often and easily?	Diabetic foot ulcers	How does the offloading requirement affect your day to day life?
	Arterial ulcers	How important is limb preservation for you?
Does the wound prevent you from being with others because of odor?		
Is the financial impact of the management of your wound impacting your life? (co-pays for home health, nutritional supplements, compression garments, enzymatic debridements or dressings, wound care center visits, etc)		

- Platelet provisional matrix recruitment—Platelets do more than just clot. They also recruit inflammatory cells to form that first matrix and produce growth factors (platelet-derived growth factors). We liken this to scaffolding in the wound that starts extracellular matrix. The necessary use of anti-platelet agents in older patients may therefore impact healing.
- Macrophages—Macrophages are smart cells that do a variety of tasks, depending on their phenotypes. Traditionally they are known as those cells that consume the pathogens. For wound healing, they regulate the cytokines in the wound. These cytokines then provide input for proliferative responses and facilitate wound closure.
- Matrix metalloproteinases (MMPs)—MMPs are enzymes that catalyze protein breakdown. They are the demolition experts in the wound. In older animal models, there may be too much of a good thing where MMPs are over-expressed and causing more inflammation and destruction.
- Fibroblasts—Where the MMPs are the demolition experts, fibroblasts are the builders.
- Growth Factors—The main growth factors discussed regarding chronic wounds are platelet-derived growth factors (PDGF) and transforming growth factor beta (TGF-B).[11,12] The growth factors impact the fibroblasts, and if there is poor response to the growth factors, there is poor wound repair.
- Extracellular matrix properties—It is important to keep in mind that older patients have skin atrophy and thinning. These properties put them not only at risk of shear, but also impair the healing overall.[13]

- Microcirculation—Too often clinicians focus on the macrocirculation, with regards to leg wounds. But it is the microcirculation that may be of higher importance, as it delivers oxygen to the wound. Abundant literature points toward the hypoxic environment in a chronic non-healing wound.[14] Delivering nutrients and removing waste products is an obvious role as well. Older skin has difficulties with vasoregulation, leading to struggles to respond to inflammation and cell production and angiogenesis.

As we have come to better understand the nature of wound healing and difficulties in older patients, we know that many wounds are "chronic" from the beginning. These wounds that disproportionately affect older adults include venous leg ulcers, arterial ulcers, pressure injuries, and diabetic foot ulcers. The combination of aging skin and underlying inflammatory responses is a recipe for preventing wound healing.

WOUND ASSESSMENT

Wound assessment does not need to be challenging, just systematic. By using a common vocabulary, providers can describe salient characteristics that help specialty wound providers triage the patient's immediate wound healing needs before they may be seen in a wound healing clinic. **Table 2** can be used as a quick reference card. When documenting the cause of the chronic wound, it is important to use the correct staging system. For instance, only pressure injuries should be staged, while diabetic foot ulcers may use the Wagner Grading System.

1. Anatomic location—Be specific. "Buttock" does not tell much about the cause of a wound as much as "right ischium" may hint at a problem with offloading when the patient is sitting.
2. Peri wound—Clues to adverse reactions to wound products or impending infection can be found in the peri wound. Skin tears can be prevented with the use of skin preparation products and adhesive removers. Contact dermatitis due to a wound product may be within 48 hours (irritant – 80% of cases) or a delayed hypersensitivity reaction and occur over weeks (allergic – 20% of cases). Use of contact allergens in skin and wound products can lend themselves to rising sensitization in patients with chronic wounds.[15] Inspect the peri wound carefully and describe any tenderness or erythema. If there is swelling or erythema, attempt to milk that area toward the wound opening in case there is a draining sinus that suggests infection.

Table 2 Wound descriptor card	
Wound Descriptor	**Details**
Anatomic location	Be specific
Peri wound	Note skin tears, dermatitis changes, tenderness
Edge	Note epithelial edge if present, maceration, cliffed, undermining
Wound bed	Differentiate between healthy viable/granulating tissue and non-viable tissue. Note any structures such as bone, tendon, ligament, or vessel. Estimate the percentage of each tissue type.
Drainage	Note quantity and color. Bright green may indicate *Pseudomonas* infection.

3. Edge—Edge effect refers to epithelialization gently sloping toward the edge. Studies suggest that those wounds with a wound edge effect have a higher chance of healing.[16] This reflects the importance of epidermal restoration discussed under chronic wounds earlier. Note whether the edge is demarcated, attached, or undermined. If the edge is cliffed or undermined, the cells will have difficulty migrating across the wound bed. Erythema extending greater than 0.5 cm from the wound can be a marker for infection, in particular with diabetic foot ulcers.[17] Maceration may be evidence of poorly controlled wound fluid management by the product chosen. Maceration can also happen due to external factors such as environment (stepping in puddles or showering without changing the wound product), or urine or feces exposure. The edge needs to be protected from this excessive moisture.

4. Wound bed—Providers should describe healthy pink granulating tissue versus nonviable tissue. Document the color, as some deep purple discoloration may indicate trauma or infection. Nonviable tissue terms include slough (wet) versus eschar (dry) and are a marker of bacterial burden.[18] Record whether there is tissue that bleeds easily, as this indicates the tissue is friable and may have a high bacterial burden. Note any structures—bone, tendon, ligament, vessel—that might be seen. Estimate the percentage of each tissue type.

5. Drainage—Ask the patient when the wound dressing was last changed. Clinical staff should date and time the dressings in order to best gauge amount of drainage at the visit. Although subjective, estimate the amount using terms such as "scant," "small,""medium," or "large." Large drainage is usually where the dressings would need to be changed daily. Also note the color—is the wound bleeding excessively or is there bright green discoloration? Bright green discoloration may indicate the presence of *Pseudomonas* bacteria in the wound because of its green pigment.

6. Size—Disposable rulers are the most cost-effective manner to measure a wound, but also may lead to inaccuracies. Wounds are not a square after all. When using rulers, it is important to measure the same way each time, sometimes noting the orientation of the body. For example, measuring a sacral pressure injury while the patient is in the right lateral decubitus position. Other measurement options include clear plastic tracing guides and computer-based imaging. Cameras with image capture and computer-based imaging are becoming more prevalent as the cost barrier has come down. This modality remains the most expensive, but emerging technology lends itself to enhanced efficiency by analyzing the edge and tissue quality and plotting healing rates over time.[19] There are also wound assessments using smartphone technology, making this a more accessible manner for clinicians.[20]

MEDICAL-LEGAL IMPLICATIONS OF WOUND CARE, AND INCORPORATION OF THE 4 M'S

As in all fields of medicine, the expectation is that the health care provider will follow evidenced-based guidelines in the care of their patient. This principle holds true for the management of acute and chronic wounds. Each type of wound, including pressure injures, venous leg ulcers, arterial wounds, and neuropathic ulcers, have treatment guidelines created by national and international wound care societies that outline appropriate wound care based on the applicable literature. Clinicians involved in wound care should be knowledgeable on the guidelines, which include not only treatment of wounds, but also proper documentation, clinical work up, and prevention strategies. Failure to follow these guidelines can result in poor outcomes, and subsequent litigation.

The acuity of the patient's wounds determines care settings. The majority of acute wounds are treated in Emergency Centers (EC]). It has been noted that of all EC malpractice claims, 5% to 20% involve wound care, with 3% to 11% of all malpractice dollars being paid for wound care-related cases.[21] Most EC cases involve retained foreign bodies, wound infections, or failure to diagnose a deeper injury to tendon or nerves. In the aging population, the most common care setting for litigation is post-acute care. Twenty-five percent of all litigation in long-term care involves wounds, with most of the medical malpractice claims in the geriatric population involving pressure injuries. In fact, pressure injuries are the second most common cause of civil suits alleging medical malpractice.[22] As in any clinical situation, communication and documentation are the cornerstones in the prevention of litigation.

Older adults are disproportionally affected by these wounds; guidelines discuss best practices without keeping in mind the Age Friendly 4M's–what Matters Most, Mobility, Medications, and Mentation. Use of the 4 M's can guide chronic wound treatment and communication with the patient and/or caregiver. For example, in some patients living with cognitive impairment, application of multi-layer compression wraps may increase agitation. An individual's difficulty understanding the need for offloading can impact their ability to heal a neuropathic foot wound on the plantar surface. Medications used for wound healing, such as collagenase, require daily dressing changes, which may be difficult for a patient with poor social support. The cost of the medication may also be prohibitive if not covered by health insurance. Mobility can significantly affect a patient's ability to offload, especially if we order offloading shoes, or place a total contact cast that will affect gait and potentially increase the risk for falls. Finally, what matters most to the patient should be upmost. An individual who is at the end of life may not want to be turned and repositioned every 2 hours to prevent or treat pressure injuries if it interferes with their sleep or causes pain at each turn. Because a holistic approach to wound care is a partnership with the patient, understanding their social, economic, and physical construct will help guide the provider in the most appropriate wound care strategies. Communicating risks and benefits and documenting the rationale of the plan of care can potentially decrease the risk of litigation.

CLINICS CARE POINTS

- Aging skin creates unique challenges in wound healing in the older adult.
- Cellular and physiologic changes in the healing cascade are impacted by the aging process.
- Be consistent and systematic in wound documentation.
- Communication and documentation are the cornerstones for decreasing the risk of litigation in chronic wound management.

DISCLOSURE

The authors have no financial affiliations or conflicts of interest.

REFERENCES

1. Fulmer T, Pelton L, editors. Age-friendly systems: a guide to using the 4ms while caring for older adults. Institute for Healthcare Improvement; 2022.
2. Mate K, Fulmer T, Pelton L, et al. Evidence for the 4Ms: interactions and outcomes across the care continuum. Aging Health 2021;7–8:469–81.

3. Levine JM. Clinical aspects of aging skin; considerations for the wound care practitioner. Adv Skin Wound Care 2020;33:12–9.
4. Tobin DJ. Introduction to skin aging. J Tissue Viability 2017;26(1):37–46.
5. Khavkin J, Ellis DA. Aging skin: histology, physiology, and pathology. Facial Plast Surg Clin N Am 2011;19:229–34.
6. Gilchrest BA, Murphy GF, Soter NA. Effect of chronologic aging and ultraviolet irradiation on Langerhans cells in human epidermis. J Invest Dermatol 1982; 79:85–8.
7. Lazarus GS, Cooper DM, Knighton DR, et al. Definitions and guidelines for assessment of wounds and evaluation of healing. Wound Repair Regen 1994; 2:165–70.
8. Gould L, Abadir P, Brem H, et al. Chronic wound repair and healing in older adults: current status and future research. JAGS 2015;63(3):427–38.
9. Carter MJ, DaVanzo J, Haught R, et al. Chronic wound prevalence and the associated cost of treatment in Medicare beneficiaries: changes between 2014 and 2019. J Med Econ 2023;26(1):894–901.
10. Shaw TJ, Martin P. Wound repair at a glance. J Cell Sci 2009;122(Pt 18):3209–13.
11. Agren MS, Steenfos HH, Dabelsteen S, et al. Proliferation and mitogenic response to PDGF-BB of fibroblasts isolated from chronic venous leg ulcers is ulcer-age dependent. J Invest Dermatol 1999;112:463–9.
12. Kim BC, Kim HT, Park SH, et al. Fibroblasts from chronic wounds show altered TGF-beta-signaling and decreased TGF-beta Type II receptor expression. J Cell Physiol 2003;195:331–6.
13. Ashcroft GS, Horan MA, Herrick SE, et al. Age-related differences in the temporal and spatial regulation of matrix metalloproteinases (MMPs) in normal skin and acute cutaneous wounds of healthy humans. CellTtissue Res. 1997;290:581–91.
14. Falanga V, Zhou L, Yufit T. Low oxygen tension stimulates collagen synthesis and COLIA1 transcription through the action of TGF-beta 1. J Cell Physiol 2002;191: 42–50.
15. Alavi A, Sibbald RG, Ladinzski B, et al. Wound-related allergic/irritant contact dermatitis. Adv Skin Wound Care 2016 Jun;29(6):278–86.
16. Falanga V, Saap LJ, Ozonoff A. Wound bed score and its correlation with healing of chronic wounds. Dermatol Ther 2006;19:383–90.
17. Lipsky BA, Senneville E, Abbas ZG, et al. Guidelines on the diagnosis and treatment of foot infection in persons with diabetes (IWGDF 2019 Update). Diabetes Metab Res Rev 2020;36(S1):e3280.
18. Schultz GS, Barrilo DJ, Mozino DW, et al. Wound bed preparation and a brief history of TIME. Int Wound J 2004 Apr;1(1):19–32.
19. Papzoglou ES, Zubkov L, Mao X, et al. Image analysis of chronic wounds for determining surface area. Wound Repair Regen 2010 Jul-Aug;18(4):349–58.
20. Wang L, Pedersen PC, Strong DM, et al. Smartphone-based wound assessment system for patients with diabetes. IEEE Trans Biomed Eng 2015;62(2):477–88.
21. Henry GL. Specific high-risk medical-legal issues. In: Henry GL, Sullivan DJ, editors. Emergency medicine risk management. Dallas: American College of Emergency Physicians; 1997. p. 475–94.
22. Fleck CA. Pressure ulcers. J Leg Nurse Consult 2012;23(1):4–14.

Wound Bed Preparation and Treatment Modalities

Wahila Alam, MD, CMS

KEYWORDS

- Wound bed preparation • Wound treatment • Wound healing • TIME

KEY POINTS

- Wound bed preparation is a systematic approach to identifying and treating the causes of delayed wound healing in chronic wounds, also known by the acronym TIME which stands for tissue, inflammation/infection, moisture balance, and edges.
- Wound dressings have been developed to target the pathophysiological state of wound being addressed, the choice of which depends on both wound and patient characteristics.
- Certain wounds are deemed non-healable, such as those where correction of blood supply is not feasible or in advanced chronic conditions and during the dying process. In such cases, the focus shifts to palliative management, that is, controlling drainage, odor, managing infection, and mitigating pain.

INTRODUCTION

Wound healing is a complex natural process to restore injured tissue. However, this process often becomes impaired resulting in failure of the wound to close in a timely manner.[1] When wounds do not follow a timely reparative process due to reasons that may include tissue hypoxia, bacterial burden, altered cellular responses and impaired collagen synthesis, and fail to close in 4 to 6 weeks, they are designated as chronic. The goal of wound bed preparation is a systematic approach to identify and remove barriers to healing by removing abnormal cells, manage bacterial load, and exudate to facilitate formation of healthy tissue.[2]

DISCUSSION

The concept of wound bed preparation was first introduced by Dr Vincent Falanga and Dr Gary Sibbald in 2000 based on their experiences with chronic wounds. Later, clinical interventions related to wound bed preparation became widely known with the acronym TIME which stands for tissue, inflammation/infection, moisture balance, and edges. Before reviewing the process of wound bed preparation, it would be

Department of Geriatrics, University of Connecticut, 263 Farmington Avenue, Farmington, CT 06030, USA
E-mail address: alam@uchc.edu

Clin Geriatr Med 40 (2024) 375–384
https://doi.org/10.1016/j.cger.2023.12.011
geriatric.theclinics.com

important to understand normal wound healing to appreciate approaches that target areas of derangement to assist wound healing.

PHASES OF WOUND HEALING

Hemostasis: This is the first stage of healing that occurs immediately after injury and lasts up to 3 hours with a goal to stop bleeding (**Fig. 1**).[3] The salient features are reflexive contraction of vascular smooth muscles causing primary vasoconstriction in response to endothelin secreted from injured endothelial cells and platelet aggregation, where platelets attach to exposed collagen in the injured endothelium and to each other forming the platelet plug. The combination of platelet aggregation and exposed endothelial cells activates Factor X, which converts prothrombin into thrombin. Thrombin in turn cleaves fibrinogen to fibrin which forms a mesh over the platelet plug to form a definitive thrombus. This serves as a provisional matrix that attracts other cells for the next stages of healing.[4]

Inflammation: Inflammation is characterized by influx of pro-inflammatory signaling proteins that flood the wound site after clot formation. This process is triggered by substances like hydrogen peroxide and cytokines (eg, interferons, interleukins, and tumor necrosis factor) produced by injured cells. The particular types of cytokines, called chemokines, are mainly responsible for migration of cells such as neutrophils and macrophages to the site of injury.[5,6] The levels of these pro-inflammatory signaling proteins are determined by bacteria, broken fibrin, and TNF-α at the wound site.

Signaled from bone marrow to the wound site, neutrophils degranulate releasing toxic granules and perform bacterial phagocytosis. Neutrophils also produce antimicrobial agents like matrix metalloproteases (MMPs) that kill bacteria and breakdown extracellular matrix (ECM) to help enter the site of injury. Once neutrophils have performed their function, their death occurs by apoptosis and then cleared by macrophages. Some subsets of neutrophils leave the wound site by a process called "reverse migration" (not by phagocytosis by macrophages). They travel through the interstitium back into the blood vessels. The clearance of neutrophils is essential in resolution of inflammation.[7] Macrophages, also signaled by chemokines, recognize, engulf, and kill pathogens and synthesize MMPs to help further break down the ECM. Macrophages mainly differ from neutrophils by their antimicrobial activity. The macrophages in the initial phase are pro-inflammatory but convert to anti-inflammatory macrophages in later stage of inflammation. The anti-inflammatory macrophages promote new blood vessel formation[8] beginning transition to granulation. In addition, macrophages signal fibroblasts to change to myofibroblasts to increase collagen production and formation of smooth muscle.

The levels of pro-inflammatory signaling proteins and neutrophils start to taper in the later half of this phase. If these substances remain at the wound site for prolonged periods, they can cause continued breakdown of growth factors and ECM resulting in secondary necrosis in the wound. Low levels of macrophages can also result in

 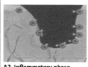 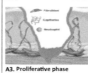

A1. Hemostasis   A2. Inflammatory phase   A3. Proliferative phase   A4. Epithelialization   A5. Maturation

Fig. 1. Phases of wound healing.

compensatory elevation in neutrophils contributing to delayed wound healing. Prolonged inflammatory phase is a common occurrence in chronic wounds.[9,10]

Granulation or proliferative phase: This phase, also known as the proliferative phase, consists of collagen formation, neovascularization, and epithelialization. Activated fibroblasts from the adjacent dermis lay down collagen to form new ECM. Some convert to myofibroblasts to help contract the wound for epithelialization.[11] Neovascularization, another integral part of this phase, starts by epithelial cells breaking away from the inner lining of blood vessels, which then sprout and branch to form new blood vessels.[12] Once the wound is completely granulated, epithelial cells proliferate from the edges, connect to each other cells by desmosomes, and close the wound. The surface epithelium then differentiates into its several layers; having its own ECM, basement membrane, cell layers, hair follicles, sebaceous and sweat glands and so forth.

Maturation: Once the wound has epithelialized and moves into maturation phase, macrophages switch to or regain their phagocytic properties. They clear unwanted cells and help with scar formation. Hyperfunction at this stage can result in skin fibrosis.[13] Wounds undergo remodeling and maturation after closing for many months or years. During this phase, collagen type III is converted to stronger and more resilient collagen type I (**Table 1**).

WOUND BED PREPARATION

Wound bed preparation is a systematic approach to identify and treat causes of delayed wound healing in a chronic wound.

Based on recent publication of Wound Bed Preparation Paradigm in 2021, the first step is to determine the healability of a wound.[14] If a wound is determined healable based on local characteristics and comorbid conditions, one would begin with local wound care including cleansing, removing slough or debridement, and managing inflammation or infection and moisture balance. Each of these steps is detailed in **Table 2**.

Cleansing: The best techniques for wound cleansing are either soaking, irrigation, or gentle pressure or massage with a goal to irrigate the wound, clear debris with care not to damage healthy tissue.[15] Flawed or incorrect technique can result in damage to healthy tissue, introduce infection, or cause maceration. The most commonly used cleanser is normal saline 0.9% which is gentle and physiologically safe. However, several antimicrobial wound cleansers such as acetic acid, chlorhexidine, povidone iodine, hydrogen peroxide, sodium hypochlorite, octenidine, and polyhexamethylene

Table 1 Phases of wound healing	
Wound Healing Phase	**Key Features**
Hemostasis	Platelet aggregation to form a clot Chemotaxis
Inflammation	Neutrophils perform phagocytosis and kill bacteria Macrophages help clear debris
Granulation	Macrophages continue to clear debris and attract fibroblasts Neovascularization Epithelialization Scar formation
Maturation	Reorganization and remodeling of collagen

Table 2
Wound assessment

Location	Essential to Identify and Document
Measurements	Length × width or surface area. Length is head to toe and width perpendicular to length or side to side
Wound base	Type of tissue, for example, necrotic, slough, or granulation
Tunneling/undermining	Describe depth or extent in o'clock manner
Wound exudate	Mild, moderate, or excessive
Drainage	Serous, sanguineous or serosanguineous, purulent
Wound edges	Clean, macerated, callused, rolled
Surrounding skin	Normal, erythematous, indurated

biguanide (PHMB) can be used when controlling bacterial overgrowth to help the wound progress toward healing.

Debridement: Clinical experience and research support wound debridement when there is slough or dead tissue.[16] The prolonged presence of slough or dead tissue in the wound bed promotes infection and persistence of pro-inflammatory cytokines prolonging the inflammatory phase of healing. Wounds with adequate blood supply should be debrided to remove dead tissue, slough, or foreign material. The method of debridement depends on local factors, availability, expertise, and whether wound is expected to heal. For example, sharp debridement would be a method of choice for healable wounds versus conservative approach for maintenance wounds or when healing is not expected.

Chronic wounds may require repeated debridement at regular intervals as slough and dead tissue may recur due to factors related to wound. It is recommended that the person performing sharp wound debridement have appropriate credentials and training to perform the task and written informed consent is always mandatory.

TYPES OF DEBRIDEMENT

Autolytic debridement uses the body's natural immune response to remove devitalized tissue with the help of specialized dressings (**Table 3**). The dressing is applied to the wound after cleansing and, depending on the type of dressing, can be left on for 2 to 3 days. This provides a moist environment to promote innate phagocytosis and endogenous enzymes (MMPs) to break down dead tissue. Some of the dressings used are hydrocolloid, calcium alginate, or hydrogel. Autolytic debridement often takes longer and relies on body's natural response which may be impaired in conditions such as diabetes, vascular disease, infection, immunodeficiency, and poor

Table 3
Types of debridement modalities

Debridement Type	Debridement Modality
Autolytic	Hydrogel, hydrocolloid
Enzymatic	Collagenase, bromelain
Sharp/excisional	Scalpel, curette, operative
Mechanical	Wet-to-dry, wet-to-moist, whirlpool, lavage
Biologic	Larval therapy
Other	Laser, ultrasound, hydrosurgery

nutritional state. Ideally if autolytic debridement takes longer than 72 hours, another form of debridement should be used.[17]

Enzymatic debridement uses an exogenous enzyme like collagenase, available in the form of a gel, to remove devitalized tissue. It has advantages over autolytic debridement as it is quicker than autolytic debridement and may play a role in reducing inflammation and promoting granulation tissue. Exogenous collagenase is known to break down denatured collagen only, thus sparing healthy tissue and making it safe to use. It is also less painful than sharp debridement.[18] Bromelain is a novel enzymatic debriding agent[19] that is derived from pineapple stems and has shown success in clinical settings including burns and chronic wounds.[20]

Sharp or excisional debridement is achieved by using a curette or scalpel to manually remove slough, devitalized, or necrotic tissue. It can be done conservatively by removing small amounts of dead tissue over several settings or extensively reaching deeper layers of the wound in single effort. Studies have shown repeated sharp debridement results in faster reduction in wound surface area and wound closure.[17,21] Debridement can be performed at the bedside, or in the operating room (OR) for larger wounds or in preparation for flap closure.

Mechanical debridement: The most common techniques used in this method are saline wet-to-dry dressing, whirlpool, or wound irrigation. Wet-to-dry dressing uses saline-soaked gauze applied to wound bed and covered with dry dressing. As the dressing dries, it adheres to necrotic tissue and pulls the tissue on removal. Wet-to-dry dressings are labor-intensive and require multiple changes in a day. This technique is painful and nonselective resulting in removal of healthy tissue and has therefore fallen out of favor. Wet-to-moist dressings can serve as a reasonable alternative. Whirlpool or irrigation is other ways of mechanical debridement. These are often unsafe as they can result in bacterial contamination or aerosolization.

Biologic debridement, also called larval therapy, uses disinfected maggots to remove necrotic tissue. Larvae of blowfly are placed on the wound that remove devitalized tissue. This method is highly effective but not widely accepted by patients and clinicians. In addition, it requires specialized settings making it difficult to access.[22]

Other debridement modalities: Hydrosurgery that uses high pressure irrigation and ultrasonic debridement has some studies supporting their use. For example, hydrosurgery may be faster than sharp debridement but not effective in all types of wounds. Laser and low-frequency ultrasonic debridement has shown promising results.[23]

Clinical pearl: For healable wounds, the most effective approach would be to start with conservative sharp debridement followed by enzymatic or autolytic debridement. This could be supplemented by periodic sharp debridement until granulation followed by moisture management until closure.

MANAGE INFECTION AND INFLAMMATION

All wounds are contaminated by microorganisms, both from native body flora and exposure to the external environment. The bacterial presence can range from contamination to colonization, critical colonization, and ultimately local and systemic infection[24] (**Table 4**).

Bacteria often adhere to the wound bed and form biofilm—a complex structure where organisms for colonies that escape the host immune cells and are less susceptible to antimicrobial treatment. The presence of biofilm causes persistent inflammatory state and delayed healing.

Based on the level of inflammation and bacterial bioburden, several interactive dressings are used to manage both. Although not backed by strong evidence, these

Table 4
Spectrum of bacterial burden of the wound

Phase	Definition
Contamination	Bacteria are present but not multiplying
Colonization	Bacteria start to multiply but do not cause host reaction
Critical colonization	Bacteria multiply, compete for nutrients, and impair wound healing Bacteria may also form biofilms
Local infection	Bacteria spread to wound and adjacent tissue causing local infection and cellulitis
Systemic infection	Bacteria spread to rest of the body causing systemic inflammatory response and sepsis

dressings offer some advantages over conventional dressings. The anti-inflammatory properties of silver and honey can help control excessive inflammation, whereas others like iodine, methylene blue, and PHMB can help with superficial infection in non-healing, foul smelling, exudative wounds that show friable granulation tissue. The decision to treat with oral or intravenous antibiotics is based on diagnosing infection and should be prescribed by a medical provider.[25,26]

MANAGE MOISTURE AND EDGES

Wounds require appropriate moisture for healing in order for cellular milieu to perform its functions. Dry wound environment can result in damage to wound bed. On the other hand, surplus moisture can result in maceration that interferes with wound healing.

Skin surrounding the wound (also known as peri-wound area) plays a vital role in wound healing. Peri-wound skin can become macerated and break down from excessive moisture. A dressing should be chosen based on whether it needs to donate or absorb moisture to the wound bed. Dressings may need to be substituted or changed based on changing moisture levels.

WOUND DRESSING TYPES

Management of chronic wounds includes both disease-specific approaches and targeted treatments (**Table 5**).[27] Wound dressings have been developed to target pathophysiological state of the wound being addressed, the choice of which depends on both wound and patient characteristics. For example, a moist occlusive dressing can support the inflammatory phase by creating a low oxygen state and wound exudate facilitating autolytic debridement. On the other hand, a semipermeable dressing like Tegaderm is used where superficial protection is needed, but at the same time, air and vapor exchange is desirable.

Both *hydrocolloid and hydrogel dressings* provide moisture balance by absorbing some fluid while maintaining a moist wound environment. Owing to this property, they are useful in autolytic debridement. Hydrogel can also provide a moist environment for dry wounds. For moderate to highly draining wounds, super absorptive dressings like alginates, derived from seaweed, can be used.

Foam dressings serve a dual purpose by their ability to absorb exudate in moderately draining wounds as well as providing moist environment for relatively dry wounds. They are favored due to their easy applicability and reduced trauma during dressing changes. Foam is often combined with anti-inflammatory or antibacterial compounds like silver and methylene blue.[28] Some dressings combine foam or other

Table 5
Wound dressings based on wound type

Wound Appearance	Types of Dressing
Necrotic	Hydrocolloid (autolytic debridement)
	Collagenase (enzymatic debridement)
	Honey
	Larval therapy
	Ultrasound
Inflamed/infected	Povidone iodine
	Silver or sulfa-containing creams
	Methylene blue/gentian violet
	Polyhexamethylene biguanide (PHMB)
	Metronidazole 1%
	Mupirocin 1%
	Acetic acid 0.5%
Draining	Alginate
	Absorbent foam
	Hydrofiber
Non-draining/dry	Transparent film
	Hydrocolloid
	Hydrogel
	Collagen gel

materials with antimicrobials to address bacterial bioburden or biofilms and assist progression to granulation and epithelialization. Care is needed in selecting appropriate antimicrobial as some like iodine are pro-inflammatory, whereas others like silver are anti-inflammatory. Gentian violet/methylene blue and PHMB are neutral and serve as good choices to manage bacterial bioburden.

Collagen dressing does not replace the collagen in the wound but works by reducing excessive protease activity during granulation, thus facilitating cell function during this phase.[29] It is used in moderately draining granulating wounds.

Specialty dressings: Engineered skin substitutes have shown promising results in difficult to heal wounds like diabetic wounds, by achieving closure within a short time compared with placebo.[30] The skin substitutes are derived from a biological source and combined with a material to be applied to a wound. For example, Dermagraft contains fibroblasts and ECM that can generate growth factors, collagen, and cytokines to promote wound healing. Disadvantages include high cost and possible hypersensitivity reactions as well as limited applicability in other types of wounds. Manufacturers claim that cost can be offset if the dressing decreases hospital length of stay.

Growth factors: Chronic wounds have decreased levels of growth factors such as platelet-derived growth factor, fibroblast growth factor, and transforming growth factor as well as IL-1, IL-6, and TNF-α. Ideally, it would make sense to address these deficiencies to promote wound healing. However, only platelet-derived growth factor has shown modest benefit in wound healing. This is available in the form a gel named becaplermin, applied directly to the wound, but cost prevents its widespread use.[31]

Negative Pressure Wound Therapy: A foam dressing attached to a suction/irrigation device ensures a moist wound environment, clears debris, promotes wound contraction, and removes exudate. There is some evidence of decreased hospital stay with the use of negative pressure wound therapy (NPWT). In many surgical wounds, NPWT is used to reduce the size of the wounds before skin grafting.[32] Systematic reviews suggest that NPWT is of benefit over standard wound therapy in achieving wound closure.

Hyperbaric oxygen therapy: Hyperbaric oxygen therapy (HBOT) requires a person to enter a chamber and inhale oxygen at two to three times higher atmospheric pressure. This results in improved tissue oxygenation, reduced hypoxia in ischemic wounds, and increased bactericidal activity. It is also thought to trigger release of growth factors thus improving leukocyte and fibroblast function and angiogenesis. HBOT is currently indicated for compromised skin grafts and flaps, necrotizing soft tissue infections, resistant osteomyelitis, and radiation osteonecrosis. HBOT has limited and low-quality evidence to support its use in ischemic and diabetic foot ulcers. Side effects include middle ear injury, temporary near sightedness, pneumothorax, and seizures.[33]

Future directions: Stem cell therapy and platelet-rich plasma have shown some promise in animal studies.[29] For example, adipose-derived mesenchymal stem cells can differentiate into various cell types such as endothelial cells, fibroblast and keratinocytes and secrete cytokines and growth factors essential for wound healing in animal models.[34–36]

SUMMARY

In conclusion, wound bed preparation is a systematic approach to wound healing in chronic wounds. It addresses factors responsible for delayed healing including excessive inflammation, necrotic tissue, high bacterial burden, infection, and moisture balance. A combination of wound debridement, specialty dressings, and advanced technologies is currently available and used successfully to facilitate the healing process. Some wounds are non-healable, for example, those where blood supply cannot be corrected, advanced comorbidities, or during the dying process. In such cases, the focus shifts to a palliative symptomatic approach, controlling drainage, odor, infection, and managing pain.

CLINICS CARE POINTS

- Determine if the wound is healable.
- Debride slough/devitalized tissue if present, using appropriate method of debridement.
- Mange inflammation and infection using appropriate local or systemic treatments.
- Manage moisture with appropriate dressings.

DISCLOSURE

None.

REFERENCES

1. Van Koppen CJ, Hartmann RW. Advances in the treatment of chronic wounds: a patent review. Expert Opin Ther Pat 2015;25(8):931–7.
2. Montandon Denys. Symposium on wound healing. Issue 3 of Clinics in plastic surgery: an international quarterly, 4. Philadelphia, Pennsylvania: W. B. Saunders Company; 1977.
3. Pool JG. Normal hemostatic mechanisms: a review. Am J Med Technol 1977;43: 776–80.
4. Furie B, Furie BC. Mechanisms of thrombus formation. N Engl J Med 2008;359: 938–49.

5. Ramesh G, MacLean AG, Philipp MT. Cytokines and chemokines at the cross-roads of neuroinflammation, neurodegeneration, and neuropathic pain. Mediat Inflamm 2013;2013:480739.

6. Martins-Green M, Petreaca M, Wang L. Chemokines and their receptors are key players in the orchestra that regulates wound healing. Adv Wound Care 2013;2: 327–47.

7. Chen WY, Rogers AA. Recent insights into the causes of chronic leg ulceration in venous diseases and implications on other types of chronic wounds. Wound Repair Regen 2007;15:434–49.

8. Leibovich SJ, Polverini PJ, Shepard HM, et al. Macrophage-induced angiogen-esis is mediated by tumour necrosis factor-alpha. Nature 1987;329:630–2.

9. Wetzler C, Kämpfer H, Stallmeyer B, et al. Large and sustained induction of che-mokines during impaired wound healing in the genetically diabetic mouse: pro-longed persistence of neutrophils and macrophages during the late phase of repair. J Invest Dermatol 2000;115:245–53.

10. Rodrigues M, Kosaric N, Bonham CA, et al. Wound healing: a cellular perspec-tive. Physiol Rev 2019;99(1):665–706.

11. Gurtner GC, Werner S, Barrandon Y, et al. Wound repair and regeneration. Nature 2008;453:314–21.

12. Eilken HM, Adams RH. Dynamics of endothelial cell behavior in sprouting angio-genesis. Curr Opin Cell Biol 2010;22:617–25.

13. Lech M, Anders HJ. Macrophages and fibrosis: how resident and infiltrating mononuclear phagocytes orchestrate all phases of tissue injury and repair. Bio-chim Biophys Acta 1832 2013;989–997.

14. Sibbald RG, Elliott JA, Persaud-Jaimangal R, et al. Wound Bed Preparation 2021. Adv Skin Wound Care 2021;34(4):183–95.

15. Rajhathy EM, Meer JV, Valenzano T, et al. Wound irrigation versus swabbing tech-nique for cleansing noninfected chronic wounds: a systematic review of differ-ences in bleeding, pain, infection, exudate, and necrotic tissue. J Tissue Viability 2023;32(1):136–43.

16. Ramundo J, Gray M. Enzymatic wound debridement. J Wound, Ostomy Cont Nurs 2008;35(3):273–80.

17. Cardinal M, Eisenbud D, Armstrong D, et al. Serial surgical debridement: a retro-spective study on clinical outcomes in chronic lower extremity wounds. Wound Repair Regen 2009;17:306–11.

18. Falanga V. Wound bed preparation and the role of enzymes: a case for multiple actions of therapeutic agents. Wounds 2002;14:47–57.

19. Shoham Y, Gasteratos K, Singer AJ, et al. Bromelain-based enzymatic burn debridement: a systematic review of clinical studies on patient safety, efficacy and long-term outcomes. Int Wound J 2023;1–20.

20. Shoham Y, Krieger Y, Tamir E, et al. Bromelain-based enzymatic debridement of chronic wounds: a preliminary report. Int Wound J 2018;15:769–75.

21. Rogers AA, Burnett S, Moore JC, et al. Involvement of proteolytic enzymes, plas-minogen activators, and matrix metalloproteinases levels in the pathology of pressure ulcers. Wound Repair Regen 1995;3:273–83.

22. Moya-López J, Costela-Ruiz V, García-Recio E, et al. Advantages of maggot debridement therapy for chronic wounds: a bibliographic review. Adv Skin Wound Care 2020;33(10):515–25.

23. Chang Y-JR, Perry J, Cross K. Low-frequency ultrasound debridement in chronic wound healing: a systematic review of current evidence. Plast Surg 2017;25:21.

24. Leaper DJ, Schultz G, Carville K, et al. Extending the TIME concept: what have we learned in the past 10 years?(*). Int Wound J 2012;9(Suppl 2):1–19.
25. Han G, Ceilley R. Chronic wound healing: a review of current management and treatments. Adv Ther 2017;34(3):599–610.
26. Sibbald RG, Elliott James A, Ayello EA, et al. Optimizing the moisture management tightrope with wound bed preparation 2015. Adv Skin Wound Care 2015; 28(10):466–76.
27. Alam W, Hasson J, Reed M. Clinical approach to chronic wound management in older adults. J Am Geriatr Soc 2021;69(8):2327–34.
28. Percival SL, Bowler P, Woods EJ. Assessing the effect of an antimicrobial wound dressing on biofilms. Wound Repair Regen 2008;16(1):52–7.
29. Cullen B, Smith R, McCulloch E, et al. Mechanism of action of PROMOGRAN, a protease modulating matrix, for the treatment of diabetic foot ulcers. Wound Repair Regen 2002;10(1):16–25.
30. Marston WA, Hanft J, Norwood P, et al. The efficacy and safety of Dermagraft in improving the healing of chronic diabetic foot ulcers: results of a prospective randomized trial. Diabetes Care 2003;26(6):1701–5.
31. Smiell JM, Wieman TJ, Steed DL, et al. Efficacy and safety of becaplermin (recombinant human platelet-derived growth factor-BB) in patients with nonhealing, lower extremity diabetic ulcers: a combined analysis of four randomized studies. Wound Repair Regen 1999;7(5):335–46.
32. Zens Y, Barth M, Bucher HC, et al. Negative pressure wound therapy in patients with wounds healing by secondary intention: a systematic review and meta-analysis of randomised controlled trials. Syst Rev 2020;9(1):238.
33. Wenhui L, Changgeng F, Lei X, et al. Hyperbaric oxygen therapy for chronic diabetic foot ulcers: an overview of systematic reviews. Diabetes Res Clin Pract 2021;176.
34. Li P, Guo X. A review: therapeutic potential of adipose-derived stem cells in cutaneous wound healing and regeneration. Stem Cell Res Ther 2018;9:302.
35. Thomas DC, Tsu CL, Nain RA, et al. The role of debridement in wound bed preparation in chronic wound: a narrative review. Ann Med Surg (Lond) 2021;71.
36. Romanelli M, Vowden K, Weir D. Exudate management made easy. Wounds Int 2010;1(2).

Pressure Injuries and Skin Failure

Jeffrey M. Levine, MD, AGSF, CWS-P[a],*,
Barbara Delmore, PhD, RN, CWCN, MAPWCA, IIWCC-NYU[b,c]

KEYWORDS

- Pressure injuries • Skin failure • Pressure injury prevention • Wound care
- Quality of care • Geriatric syndromes • Pressure injury treatment

KEY POINTS

- Pressure injuries are associated with multiple adverse outcomes including increased length of stay, increased chance of hospital readmission within 30 days, increased risk of placement in a skilled nursing facility, increased costs of care, prolonged rehabilitation, pain, disfigurement, infection, loss of limb, and death.
- Because of their association with the perception and measurement of quality, pressure injuries have become an important concern in regulatory, reimbursement, and risk management arenas.
- Most pressure injuries are preventable through individualized and strategic prevention strategies that include positioning of vulnerable areas, moisture management, pressure redistribution surfaces, and offloading devices. However, there are nonmodifiable intrinsic risk factors that can lead to pressure injuries even when appropriate prevention strategies are diligently applied.
- Some pressure injuries may be component of the clinical syndrome of skin failure or as unavoidable consequence of skin changes at the end of life. There is currently no consensus as to whether skin failure is a separate entity from pressure injury.

INTRODUCTION

Pressure injuries have long been recognized as a consequence of illness and immobility. In the sixteenth century Ambrose Paré, considered the father of modern surgery, described healing a pressure ulcer in a soldier debilitated by the wounds of war.[1] As the director of the Saltpêtrière Hospital in nineteenth century Paris, Jean Martin Charcot proposed the first classification of pressure injuries, including *decubitus acutus* that occurs with neurologic injury, *decubitus chronicus* in debilitated persons, and

[a] Department of Geriatric Medicine and Palliative Care, Icahn School of Medicine at Mount Sinai, NY 10010, USA; [b] Center for Innovations in the Advancement of Care, Departments of Nursing, NYU Langone Health, 1 Park Avenue, 3rd Floor, Room 322, NY 10016, USA; [c] Hansjörg Wyss, Department of Plastic Surgery, NYU Grossman School of Medicine
* Corresponding author.
E-mail address: jlevinemd@shcny.com

Clin Geriatr Med 40 (2024) 385–395
https://doi.org/10.1016/j.cger.2023.12.006
0749-0690/24/© 2024 Elsevier Inc. All rights reserved.

geriatric.theclinics.com

decubitus ominosus where death is expected.[2] The incidence and prevalence of pressure injuries increased dramatically in the latter part of the twentieth century with the aging demographic and advances in medical technology that enabled people to live longer with multiple comorbidities.

A pressure injury is a chronic wound that occurs across all health care settings including hospital, skilled nursing, and home care and is associated with adverse outcomes including pain, infection, increased cost, prolonged rehabilitation, disfigurement, amputations, and mortality. Pressure injuries increase the risk for skilled nursing facility placement and rehospitalization within 30 days. They have major quality of life consequences including social isolation, financial hardship, anxiety, depression, and mobility limitations that require environmental adaptations. It is estimated that the cost of pressure injuries in US hospitals alone could exceed $26.8 billion.[3]

According to the National Pressure Injury Advisory Panel (NPIAP), pressure injury is defined as localized damage to the skin and/or underlying tissue, usually over a bony prominence that results from pressure or pressure in combination with shear.[4] Pressure injuries can be partial- or full-thickness wounds. The staging system defined by NPIAP is reserved only for pressure injuries (**Fig. 1**). Staging of pressure injuries is determined by visible depth, and if the base of the wound cannot be seen due to slough and/or eschar, the wound is determined as unstageable. A wound is designated a deep tissue pressure injury (DTPI) when the skin is intact and/or a blood-filled blister is present with purple, maroon, or bruise-like discoloration to an area subjected to pressure. A DTPI tends to evolve into a full-thickness wound including hallmark characteristics of epidermal separation, slough and/or eschar (unstageable), and/or an ulceration (Stages 3 and 4). Less commonly, a DTPI can also become a partial-thickness wound or resolve without tissue loss—a mechanism not well understood.[5,6] Medical device-related pressure injuries (MDRPIs) are caused by devices such as oxygen tubing and masks, urinary catheters, tracheostomy tubes, compression stockings, orthopedic braces, and other devices that are an integral part of care in health care settings (**Fig. 2**).

Pressure Injury Assessment

The standard skin assessment to detect the presence of a pressure injury includes a visual and tactile, head-to-toe process particularly paying attention over the bony prominences. The visual assessment observes for areas of discoloration, whereas the tactile assessment looks for areas of possible damage such as bogginess or firmness. If the individual can verbalize, the assessment process also relies on determining if any areas are causing pain.[5] Along with the visual/tactile skin assessment, a patient's risk for developing a pressure injury is calculated by using a risk assessment instrument such as the Braden Scale, which measures intrinsic and extrinsic factors that predispose to pressure injury formation.[5]

Skin and risk assessments should be performed regularly, and the timing of assessments is based on location in the health care continuum—hospital, long term care (LTC) facility, outpatient clinic, or home setting. For example, in a hospital or LTC setting, skin and risk assessments are performed on admission, daily, deterioration, and discharge. In an outpatient clinic setting, a skin and risk assessment is performed at each visit. The goal of performing skin and risk assessments at regular intervals is to ensure that the skin is free from any pressure damage, and based on the individual's risk for developing a pressure injury, timely individualized prevention strategies are implemented.[5]

It is well-known that dark skin tones impact the ability to detect Stage 1 pressure injuries and DTPIs, as increased melanocytes and other chromophores will mask the appearance of discoloration that marks the beginning phases of wound genesis

PRESSURE INJURY STAGING
Images copyright © JM Levine 2016

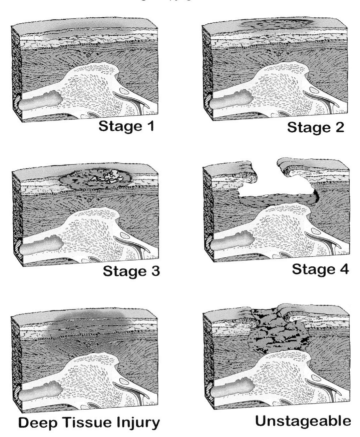

Stage 1   **Stage 2**

Stage 3   **Stage 4**

Deep Tissue Injury   **Unstageable**

Fig. 1. Pressure injuries are staged from 1 to 4 depending on depth visualized. Deep tissue pressure injury (DTPI) is a maroon or bruise-like discoloration to an area subjected to pressure, whereas the term unstageable is used when the base of the wound cannot be visualized. (*Courtesy of* Jeffrey M. Levine MD, AGSF, CWS-P.)

(**Fig. 3**). Melanin in the epidermis can mask discoloration associated with pressure injuries such as redness, purple, maroon, and blue. In such cases, these colors may present more as hyperpigmentation rather than actual injury. Assessment should be performed with adequate lighting and supplemented by palpation of potentially disrupted areas, as pressure injury can be accompanied by blistering, warmth, and induration.[7]

The most common pressure injury sites are the sacrococcygeal and heel areas. This is largely due to the altered circulation to these areas in combination with pressure due to prolonged immobility.[8,9] Although pressure injuries notably appear over bony prominences, they can occur in other anatomic areas due to medical devices or anywhere that an external pressure source comes in contact with the skin. A severe pressure injury can occur when an older adult falls at home and is down for several hours before discovered. In this case, the pressure source may be a tub, radiator, or door. Regardless of

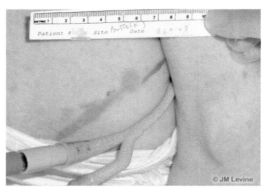

Fig. 2. This is a medical device-related pressure injury (MDRPI) from a urinary catheter imprinted onto the thigh.

location, all pressure injuries are staged according to the NPIAP or the European Pressure Ulcer Advisory Panel pressure injury/ulcer staging system.[4,5] Note that the term MDRPI is not a stage rather a description for pressure injury causation. In this case, the pressure injury is staged using the NPIAP classification system.[4]

Mucosal Membrane Pressure Injuries occur when a device (eg, endotracheal tube, Foley catheter) causes pressure to the mucosa. Pressure injuries on mucosal areas cannot be staged using the NPIAP staging system because the histology of the mucous membranes varies greatly from skin and underlying tissues.[4]

There are two caveats when staging pressure injuries. Never stage a pressure injury when the wound bed is not visualized due to eschar and/or slough. In these instances, pressure injuries are termed unstageable. Never downstage a full-thickness pressure injury as it heals such as from Stage 4 to 3. This is because full-thickness layers such as subcutaneous, muscle, tendon, cartilage, and bone do not regenerate. Rather the defect heals with granulation or scar tissue, which is only approximately as 80% strong as the original full-thickness layers.[10] As these ulcers heal, they are termed

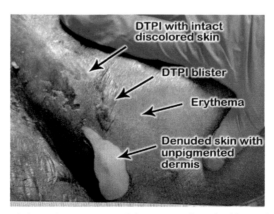

Fig. 3. Sacrococcygeal deep tissue pressure injury. Note that the blister does not display the typical purple, maroon, and bluish discoloration seen on light skin tones. The area of erythema is difficult to see as well. The area of denuded dark skin reveals exposed dermis. (*Courtesy of* Barbara Delmore PhD, RN, CWCN, MAPWCA, IIWCC-NYU, FAAN.)

healing or healed Stage 4 or 3. It is important to note that a healed Stage 4 or 3 pressure injury are susceptible to recurring due to the presence of scar tissue and when an individual possesses intrinsic or is exposed to extrinsic risk factors.[5] Such a wound is termed *recidivistic*.[11]

Documentation of pressure injury assessment is an important and essential component of care. Clear and comprehensive documentation is also a communication mechanism to all clinicians caring for the individual conveying the status of the wound. Comprehensive documentation includes stage, location, measurement (length, width, and depth in centimeters), presence of odor and/or drainage, presence of undermining and tunneling, and characteristics of the wound bed, margin, and surrounding (periwound) skin. Supplemental information includes warmth, capillary refill, and presence of pulses, edema, anasarca, and lymphedema.

Measurement is an important parameter, particularly when determining effectiveness of clinical interventions or extent of healing or deterioration. Measurement involves head-to-toe length, width, and depth and should be consistent and accurate. The simplest method uses a centimeter ruler to measure length and width, and a cotton-tipped swab to measure depth, tunneling, and undermining. Many wounds have variable appearance. If a wound is a pressure injury and the stage cannot be determined, the clinician should describe the wound in narrative form until the time it can be staged. Pressure injuries should be listed as a problem in physician notes and addressed with a nutritional evaluation and timely consultation from wound care nurses or other specialist trained in wound care.

Pressure Injury Prevention

Prevention strategies are critical for preventing pressure injuries. Based on an individual's risk factors, strategies should be individualized and tailored to their care needs. Typical prevention involves a multifaceted assessment and process.[5] Once the pressure injury risk for an individual has been determined, prevention strategies include offloading devices such as heel-lift boots, turning wedges, and pressure redistribution surfaces such as overlays, mattresses, procedure table pads, and seating cushions. It is cautioned that only commercially produced devices be used to properly offload or redistribute pressure, as "homemade" devices can cause pressure injuries because they lack appropriate redistributing or offloading properties required for proper prevention.[5]

It is recommended that interventions are "bundled" as a means to provide targeted, standard, and consistent pressure injury prevention measures.[12] A typical bundle may include selected prevention measures based on patient needs. Examples of interventions that may be included in a bundle are.

- Skin and risk assessment
- Skin care and products
- All types of pressure redistribution support surfaces
- Offloading devices and practices
- Nutrition and hydration measures
- Turning and repositioning techniques
- Patient, family, and clinician training

Although bundles are targeted measures, all recommended prevention modalities should be present in a facility's comprehensive pressure injury prevention model. Careful attention to guidelines, procedures, policies, and protocols are equally important including regular updates based on the latest evidence.

It is important to note that it is everyone's job to mitigate pressure injury formation regardless of their role in a facility. To that end, clinicians and other interprofessional team members should receive education through a variety of venues regularly and as needed. Education extends to the patient, family, caregivers, and significant others so that they are aware and understand the prevention plan. They should also be afforded the opportunity to participate in the plan's development.

Products that support skin health should be applied at regular intervals (at least twice daily and as needed) and are readily available for staff to use. In particular, there are products that provide a "barrier" on the skin of an at-risk individual to protect the skin against the caustic effects of urine and feces which raise the skin's pH, thereby making it vulnerable.[13] Offloading devices ensure that the skin is protected from pressure sources. Devices are available to assist with turning and repositioning as well as offloading heels.[5,9]

Optimization of nutrition and hydration should be considered part of the prevention process. Malnutrition and dehydration render an individual vulnerable to pressure injury formation.[5,14] Nutritional recommendations should be individualized in response to clinical conditions and goals of care, as opposed to rigidly set guidelines. The current recommendation is to assess an individual's risk using a validated nutritional risk screening instrument.[5] Along with assessing risk, other factors should be considered such as.

- History of weight loss
- Presence of dysphagia
- Current daily intake
- Anthropometric parameters including height, weight, and body mass index

Malnutrition occurs due to inadequate intake of macro- and micronutrients or the inability to absorb and metabolize nutrients. Therefore, clinicians should be vigilant to assess for comorbidities and conditions that contribute to malnutrition including malabsorption. If an individual is considered at high risk for pressure injury formation and/or malnourished, recommendations include a diet consisting of.

- 30 to 35 calories/kg/day
- 1.2 to 1.5 g/kg body weight/day of protein intake
- 50% to 60% carbohydrates
- 20% to 25% fats
- 1 mL of fluid intake per kcal/day

In addition, vitamin and mineral supplements should be included as indicated.[5,14,15]

Redistribution surfaces are important in the prevention and treatment of pressure injuries. Low-air-loss (LAL) technologies provide pressure redistribution, microclimate support and, for some patients, decrease pain and increase comfort. Facilities should evaluate all the possible areas that redistribution surfaces (eg, mattresses, overlays), table pads, and seating cushions are necessary, and regularly inspect these surfaces so that they are replaced as needed.[5]

Durable medical equipment (DME) for pressure redistribution is essential for preventing pressure injuries. The terms "Group 1" and "Group 2" are often used to categorize different types of support surfaces or mattresses. These classifications are set by the Centers for Medicare and Medicaid Services (CMS) and are associated with reimbursement codes used in billing and insurance claims. The main differences between Group 1 and Group 2 DME devices for pressure injury prevention are in their features, complexity, and intended use.

Group 1 DME includes basic support surfaces, such as standard mattresses and overlays, which are primarily designed for comfort and pressure distribution but may not have advanced features. These support surfaces are usually static, meaning they do not have moving or alternating components to actively change pressure points. They redistribute pressure passively by using materials like foam or other cushioning. Group 1 DME devices are generally more affordable and suitable for patients with lower risk or partial-thickness pressure injuries.

Group 2 DME includes more advanced support surfaces, such as alternating pressure mattresses, LAL mattresses, air-fluidized beds, and kinetic therapy beds. These support surfaces are dynamic and have components that actively change pressure distribution. Alternating pressure mattresses, for example, inflate and deflate cells to periodically shift the patient's weight, reducing pressure on specific areas. Group 2 DME devices are typically more expensive than Group 1 devices and are used for patients at higher risk of pressure injuries or those with existing pressure ulcers.

Pressure relief and/or pressure redistribution devices should be applied in accordance with an individualized plan consistent with patient assessment, facility policies, and clinical practice guidelines. Other types of pressure redistribution and relieving devices include specialized seat cushions, heel and elbow protectors, positioning devices such as wedges and rolls, wheelchair seating systems, and transfer aids used for repositioning. Most of these are classified as Group 1 DME. Depending on the device, they may only provide pressure relief, not pressure redistribution. Pressure relief focuses on actively relieving pressure on specific body areas at risk of developing pressure injuries through repositioning and offloading techniques, whereas pressure redistribution involves using specialized equipment and surfaces to evenly distribute pressure across the body's surface, reducing the overall risk of pressure injuries. Both strategies are essential components of pressure injuries prevention and management in health care settings.

Treatment of Pressure Injuries

Treatment relies on establishing the etiology of a wound so that the specific cause can be addressed. Stage-based treatment of pressure injuries, once a standard of care, is now considered obsolete. The same prevention strategies that are used to prevent pressure injuries (eg, support surfaces, offloading devices, turning, and positioning) are used to help heal a pressure injury. Treatment decisions are multifactorial and include patient-centered concerns and nutritional status as well as wound bed characteristics.[16] A comprehensive, systematic evaluation of the patient and underlying medical conditions should be used before implementing a treatment plan.

Before treating any wound, goals for healing should be addressed. If healing is the goal, the wound bed is assessed, and the appropriate topical treatment (dressing) is applied to help heal the wound.[16] A variety of topical treatments are available in different categories designed to match the wound bed characteristics intended to be addressed and foster healing. Basic categories include products that donate moisture, remove excessive moisture, provide antimicrobial action, and debride. Some products are designed to address shallow wounds, whereas other products are useful for filling cavities, undermining, and tunneling. Some wounds require excisional debridement to remove dead tissue and allow topical treatment to be effective.

Wound bed preparation is a crucial aspect of wound care and management that involves a systematic and comprehensive approach to creating an optimal environment for wound healing.[16] The patient and their circle of caregivers should be included through all steps of the management approach. The approach encompasses various actions and strategies to facilitate the healing process by addressing the condition of the wound bed. Proper wound bed preparation helps reduce the risk of infection, promotes tissue regeneration, and accelerates the healing process. Elements of wound bed preparation include.

- Assessment
- Removal of dead or infected tissue (debridement)
- Management of infection
- Moisture balance
- Protection and promotion of newly formed tissue
- Pain management
- Patient/family education

Debridement methods include surgical debridement, mechanical debridement (using dressings or irrigation), enzymatic debridement, and autolytic debridement (allowing the body's natural processes to remove dead tissue).

Numerous wound care products are available; however, there is variable evidence regarding their efficacy. Part of the reason is due to U.S. Food and Drug Administration (FDA) classifications of most wound care products as "medical devices" as opposed to pharmaceuticals, which exempt manufacturers from the requirement to produce data supporting effectiveness. With limited evidence-based support for products, choices are often made based on availability, cost considerations, expert opinion, and intrinsic rationale for product type.

Palliative Care for Pressure Injuries

Palliative care for pressure injuries should be considered when it becomes clear that there is little or no realistic chance of healing within the patient's lifetime and when the burdens of operative procedures or advanced treatment options outweigh the benefits.[17] Factors leading to designating a wound as palliative include unmodifiable risk factors or medical conditions such as malnutrition with sarcopenia, inadequate perfusion, multisystem organ failure, immunocompromise, anasarca, metastatic cancer, and a terminal prognosis that prevents the normal healing process. A palliative approach can reduce suffering, improve quality of life, and decrease health care costs by eliminating futile and/or painful procedures and treatments, and curtail unnecessary health care costs.

The decision to designate a wound as palliative arises when the wound is unresponsive to therapy and the process of achieving healing is inconsistent with goals of care. Some pressure injuries designated as palliative can show signs of healing, but this should not alter the overall plan. A palliative approach may include modification of timing of dressings and repositioning to decrease pain associated with physical manipulation of the patient and the wound. Topical pain treatments include viscous lidocaine gel and dressings that deliver locally applied ibuprofen and opiates. Wound odor can be minimized with charcoal- or chlorophyll-containing dressings, antiseptics, ionized silver dressings, or metronidazole gel[OL]. Dressings such as alginates, hydrofibers, and absorptive foam dressings can manage excess drainage and protect the periwound areas from moisture associated skin damage (MASD).

Skin Failure and Unavoidable Pressure Injury

Although the occurrence of pressure injury has been closely linked with quality of care, it is increasingly recognized that pressure injuries can occur when all clinical practice guidelines for prevention have been followed. The term "skin failure" has been proposed to account for unavoidable pressure injury. Like all other organs skin can fail; however, experts continue to grapple with definitions, causative factors, and manifestations.[18] A comprehensive definition of skin failure is the state in which tissue tolerance is so compromised that cells can no longer survive in zones of physiologic impairment that includes hypoxia, local mechanical stresses, impaired delivery of nutrients, and buildup of toxic metabolic byproducts.[19]

Several authors have proposed a variety of terminologies and clinical syndromes which fall within the spectrum of skin failure. These include the Kennedy Terminal Ulcer, Trombley-Brennan terminal tissue injury, skin failure at life's end, and acute skin failure.[18] A key to understanding skin failure is acknowledging the physiologic factors that act synergistically to cause unavoidable skin injury.[19] These include, but may not be limited to, sarcopenia, malnutrition, hypoxia, poor perfusion related to low output states, edema, inflammation, increased vascular permeability, systemic inflammatory response syndrome, multiple organ system failure, metastatic disease, and physiologic changes associated with the dying process. Unlike other organ systems there is currently no laboratory marker identifying skin failure, and universal agreement on its definition has not yet been reached. Clinicians should determine whether a wound may be a manifestation of skin failure through critical questioning regarding the primary etiology of the wound (eg, hypoperfusion vs pressure).[19]

Medical-Legal Aspects of Pressure Injuries

Pressure injuries have a long-standing association with the perception and measurement of quality. There is a growing trend among personal injury and medical malpractice attorneys to bring litigation against facilities and health care workers when facility-acquired pressure injuries and related complications have ensued. Such claims received increased traction with CMS designation of hospital-acquired pressure injuries as a potentially nonreimbursable event and published studies correlating inadequate staffing levels with occurrence of new wounds.[20] Commonly claimed damages include pain, suffering, scarring and disfigurement, infection, amputation, and cause of death. According to the Agency for Healthcare Research and Quality, more than 17,000 lawsuits related to pressure injuries are filed annually.

In pursuing such claims, facilities are held to national standards published in clinical practice guidelines as well as local standards outlined in each facility's policy and procedure manual. Long-term care facilities face the challenge of compliance with standards set in Federal Tag 686 which comprises detailed guidelines for surveyors.[21] Photographs of wounds embedded within the medical record or taken by concerned family members add to the shock value of litigation claims when presented to a lay jury. Other factors that contribute to the value of pressure injury litigation include the lack of wound care education in medical training with leaves many primary care physicians with limited knowledge of prevention, assessment, and treatment for pressure injuries.

SUMMARY

The older adult is vulnerable to pressure injury formation due to the associated skin changes and multimorbidities.[5] Preventing and treating pressure injuries are complex processes. More importantly, these processes require an interprofessional approach. Clinical team members, the patient, and their circle of caregivers should have input and an understanding of the goals of care.[17] Both prevention and treatment approaches should be based on the latest evidence and comprehensive. The cost of treating a pressure injury far outweighs the costs associated with evidence-based prevention practices. All care should be targeted to prevent or expeditiously treat a pressure injury to avoid the consequences of poor wound-related outcomes.[3]

CLINICS CARE POINTS

- All pressure injuries should be examined and documented by the primary care physician and added to the active problem list.
- If the wound could not be prevented (ie, refusals, multiple organ system disease, end of life, skin failure) write a narrative note explaining your clinical thought process and rationale.
- Nutritional interventions with proper intake of protein, calories, and micronutrients are key components of pressure injury prevention and treatment.
- Classic signs and symptoms of infection may be absent in older adults or persons with diabetes or immune compromise.
- For wounds with little to no chance of healing, use a palliative approach with symptom management. Work with surgical specialists and counsel patients and their circle of care givers to limit aggressive measures, and document your efforts.

DISCLOSURE

The authors have no financial disclosures.

REFERENCES

1. Levine JM. Historical notes on pressure ulcers: the cure of Ambrose Paré. Decubitus 1992;5:23–6.
2. Levine JM. Historical perspective: the neurotrophic theory of skin ulceration. J Am Geriatr Soc 1992;12:1281–3.
3. Padula WV, Delarmente BA. The national cost of hospital-acquired pressure injuries in the United States. Int Wound J 2019;2018:1–7.
4. Edsberg LE, Black JM, Goldberg M, et al. Revised national pressure ulcer advisory panel pressure injury staging system. journal of wound. Ostomy and Continence Nursing 2016;43(6):585–97.
5. European Pressure Ulcer Advisory Panel, National Pressure Injury Advisory Panel, Pan Pacific Pressure Injury Alliance. Prevention and Treatment of Pressure Ulcers/Injuries: Clinical Practice Guideline. The International Guideline. (Haesler E, ed.). European Pressure Ulcer Advisory Panel, National Pressure Injury Advisory Panel and Pan Pacific Pressure Injury Alliance; 2019.
6. Tescher AN, Thompson SL, McCormack HE, et al. A retrospective, descriptive analysis of hospital-acquired deep tissue injuries. Ostomy Wound Manage 2018;64(11):30–41.
7. Black J, Cox J, Capasso V, et al. Current perspectives on pressure injuries in persons with dark skin tones from the national pressure injury advisory panel. Adv Skin Wound Care 2023;36(9):470–80.
8. Delmore B, Sprigle S, Samim M, et al. Does sacrococcygeal skeletal morphology and morphometry influence pressure injury formation in adults? Adv Skin Wound Care 2022;35(11):586–95.
9. Delmore B, Ayello EA, Smith D, et al. Refining heel pressure injury risk factors in the hospitalized patient. Adv Skin Wound Care 2019;32(11):512–9.
10. Marshall CD, Hu MS, Leavitt T, et al. Cutaneous scarring: basic science, current treatments, and future directions. Adv Wound Care 2018;7(2):29–45.
11. Tew C, Hettrick H, Holden-Mount S, et al. Recurring pressure ulcers: identifying the definitions. a national pressure ulcer advisory panel white paper. Wound Repair Regen 2014;22(3):301–4.

12. Garcia AD, Delmore B, Capasso V, et al. Challenges in the prevention and treatment of pressure injuries. Health Europa 2022.

13. Nguyen AV, Soulika AM. The dynamics of the skin's immune system. Int J Mol Sci 2019;20(8):1–54.

14. Munoz N, Litchford M, Cox J, et al. National pressure injury advisory panel white paper malnutrition and pressure injury risk in vulnerable populations: application of 2019 International Clinical Practice Guideline. Adv Skin Wound Care 2022; 35(March):156–65.

15. Posthauer ME, Dorner B, Chu AS. Nutrition and wound care. In: Baranoski S, Ayello EA, editors. Wound care essentials: practice principles. 5th edition. Philadelphia, PA: Chapter 10. Wolters Kluwer; 2020. p. 242–69.

16. Sibbald RG, Elliott JA, Persaud-Jaimangal R, et al. Wound bed preparation 2021. Adv Skin Wound Care 2021;34(4):183–95.

17. Beers EH. Palliative wound care: less is more. Surg Clin 2019;99:899–919.

18. Ayello EA, Levine JM, Langemo D, et al. Reexamining the literature on terminal ulcers, scale, skin failure, and unavoidable pressure injuries. Adv Skin Wound Care 2019;32(3):109–21.

19. Levine JM, Delmore B, Cox J. Skin failure: concept review and proposed model. Adv Skin Wound Care 2022;35(3):139–48.

20. Centers for Medicare & Medicaid Services (CMS). HHS. Medicare program: changes to the hospital inpatient prospective payment systems and fiscal year 2008 rates. Fed Regist 2007;72(162):47129–8175. PubMed: 17847578.

21. Centers for Medicare & Medicaid Services. Requirements for Long-Term Care Facilities, F-Tag 686 Skin Integrity. Available at https://www.cms.gov/Medicare/Provider-Enrollment-and-Certification/GuidanceforLawsAndRegulations/Nursing-Homes. Accessed August 7, 2023.

Arterial Leg Ulcers in the Octogenarian

Allegra L. Fierro, MD[a],*, Marnie Abeshouse, MD[a],
Tomer Lagziel, MD[a], John C. Lantis II, MD[a,b,1]

KEYWORDS

- Arterial leg ulcers • Geriatric leg ulcers • Adjunctive therapies for ischemic disease

KEY POINTS

- Arterial leg ulcer (ALU) management in the octogenarian highlights the multifaceted challenges inherent in geriatric medicine and vascular surgery, and a multimodal management approach is essential.
- Adjunctive devices and tissue-based therapies can greatly benefit ALU healing regardless of revascularization when used with standard of care (SOC).
- Although revascularization remains the primary way to assure that patients heal arterial ulcers even in the octogenarian, the inherent risks of revascularization must be considered in this fragile population.

THE PROBLEM WITH GERIATRIC ARTERIAL LEG ULCERS

More than 200 million adults are affected by peripheral arterial disease (PAD) globally, and its prevalence continues to increase in the geriatric population at an alarming rate, affecting more than 29% of male and female octogenarians equally.[1] PAD exists on a clinical spectrum, with early PAD frequently remaining asymptomatic and ALUs representing end-stage disease. When an ALU manifests from severe arterial-occlusive disease, a patient is deemed to have critical limb-threatening ischemia (CLTI; **Fig. 1**).

CLTI, defined as severe PAD with associated rest pain or tissue loss, is diagnosed in only 10% to 12% of those with PAD; however, among those afflicted, CLTI drastically affects patient functional status and quality of life (QOL) and exponentially increases the likelihood of future amputation, morbidity, and death, regardless of age.[2] The 5-year mortality after an ALU diagnosis is noted as high as 55%.[3] In the octogenarian, a diagnosis of CLTI frequently represents a terminal event because the pathophysiology

[a] Department of Surgery, Icahn School of Medicine at Mount Sinai, One Gustave L. Levy Place, New York, NY 10029, USA; [b] Department of Surgery, Mount Sinai West, 425 West 59th Street, 7th Floor, New York, NY 10019, USA
[1] Senior Author
* Corresponding author.
E-mail address: Allegra.Fierro@mountsinai.org

Clin Geriatr Med 40 (2024) 397–411
https://doi.org/10.1016/j.cger.2023.12.010
0749-0690/24/© 2024 Elsevier Inc. All rights reserved.

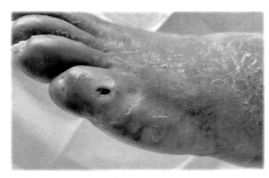

Fig. 1. Distal ischemic ulcer in octogenarian.

of the disease coupled with comorbidities and predisposing risk factors negatively affect outcomes regardless of intervention.[4]

Several risk factors that predispose to atherosclerotic disease also affect progression and prognosis in those with PAD. Smoking quadruples the likelihood of developing PAD, and more than 70% of patients with CLTI are current or former smokers. At 10 years, cardiovascular mortality in smokers with CLTI is 3 times that in nonsmokers.[5] Diabetes mellitus (DM) also quadruples the risk of developing CLTI and is a poor prognostic indicator. The likelihood of amputation is 5 times higher, and mortality is 3 times higher in patients with a dual diagnosis of DM and PAD.[6]

Coupled with decreased functional status, poor nutrition, and lack of social support, once an ALU develops, there is a high risk for progression to a chronic or nonhealing state, increasing the risk for infection, gangrene, amputation, and death. ALUs represent a significant health concern, and a multidisciplinary treatment approach geared to address symptoms, minimize complications, optimize comorbidities, and improve QOL is paramount.[7]

NONINTERVENTIONAL OPTIONS

Several noninterventional therapies have emerged during the last few decades for managing patients with chronic, nonhealing ischemic ulcers. Owing to the pathophysiology underlying PAD, most tend to fall short of revascularization when it comes to an ALU and function mainly as adjunctive measures. However, when used as part of a multimodal management plan, some of these options have facilitated ALU healing in patients who are not candidates for revascularization. In the octogenarian, these adjunctive approaches can be essential in the armamentarium for wound management, and understanding their benefits, limitations, and indications are of utmost importance.

Devices

Arterial counterpulsation

Intermittent pneumatic compression (IPC) is a well-recognized method for improving circulation. IPC is best known for its application in the inpatient setting as venous thromboembolism (VTE) prophylaxis. Although less clinically recognized, IPC is also a highly effective treatment alternative for patients with critical limb ischemia who are not candidates for intervention.

IPC involves rapid, sequential pneumatic cuff inflations and deflations that alter hemodynamics and improve arterial perfusion. It must be noted that this can be quite uncomfortable for some patients, to the point that discomfort precludes therapy. This improved perfusion is theorized to result from 3 interplaying mechanisms, the most important of which is the development of an increased arteriovenous pressure gradient. As a pneumatic cuff inflates around the limb to a pressure that is ideally close to systolic, venous pressure increases, and venous return is promoted to the heart, causing a transient decrease in the venous pressure in the limb. This transiently increased pressure gradient promotes improved arterial inflow. Second, IPC promotes shear stress-induced endothelial nitric oxide release, directly vasodilating and decreasing peripheral resistance to improve inflow. Finally, IPC is thought to temporarily suspend the venoarteriolar reflex by preventing baroreceptor stretch, as reflex vasoconstriction is inhibited without stretch.[8]

IPC has shown promise in patients with CLTI, although data has been limited to mainly clinical outcomes and case series. One prospective parallel-controlled study in patients with CLTI found that peak walking time, wound surface area, and pain improved significantly in 18 patients after 6 months of IPC compared with the 16 controls who followed an unsupervised exercise regimen.[9] Similar findings were noted in an randomized controlled trial (RCT) that included 34 inoperable patients with CLTI or PVD randomized to undergo either IPC or exercise. After 16 weeks, wound area reduced by 71% in the IPC group compared with 56% in the control group, and peak walking time ($P = .043$), pain ($P = .038$), and QOL ($P < .05$) all significantly improved after IPC compared with controls.[10]

An additional retrospective analysis published in 2016 showed that among 187 patients who were prescribed IPC, toe pressures significantly increased ($P = .071$) and rest pain significantly decreased ($P < .0001$) in those who used obtained and used device (81.72% of patients) after a median of 4 months of use. A slight reduction in minor amputation and amputation-free survival ($P = .023$, $P = .01$) was also noted.[11]

Although these studies unquestionably demonstrate that IPC can be an effective postrevascularization adjunct in patients with ALUs, the lack of large, well-controlled, and randomized trials has prevented IPC from receiving significant insurance coverage, and its use has been cost-prohibitive for many. To consider the true benefit of IPC for healing ALUs, pain reduction, and overall amputation-free survival, significantly more clinical evidence is needed.

Low-intensity ultrasound

Ultrasound (US) is considered a diagnostic gold standard for vascular disease. The use of US as a therapeutic modality for vascular disease is a newer, more controversial concept. It has been proposed that mechanical vibrations and low-frequency, low-intensity ultrasound (LIS) alter cell membrane signaling pathways to promote collagen and growth factor production and induce angiogenesis.[12]

During recent years, several studies have also demonstrated the efficacy of LIS in healing chronic wounds, including ALUs. One open-label RCT by Kavros and colleagues randomized 70 patients with nonhealing lower extremity ulcers from CLTI to undergo either LIS therapy with standard wound care or standard wound care alone, and after 12 weeks, 63% of patients in the treatment group had greater than 50% reduction in wound area size compared with 29% in the control ($P < .001$).[9]

In another notable yet small study by Yusoff and colleagues, 14 patients with non-revascularizable CLTI were treated with LIS (mean LIS exposure was 381 ± 283 days), and rates of major amputation and death were followed. After 5 years, the overall amputation-free survival rate was significantly higher in patients treated with LIS than the controls (3 vs 14). No significant difference was seen in mortality.[13]

Despite these promising findings, more clinical evidence is needed before conclusions can be definitively made about the benefits of LIS in patients with ALUs.

Electrostimulation

Electrical flow in the body is essential to proper physiologic functioning, and when electrical currents and potentials are inadequate or absent, various systems fail, and pathology can ensue. Among these systems, the skin relies on a current generated between the epidermal and subepidermal layers, called the transepithelial potential (TEP), to facilitate wound healing. When a wound develops, the TEP is interrupted, and a cascade of cellular events is triggered to restore the TEP and heal the wound.[14] In a chronic wound, the local inflammatory environment affects cellular and molecular mechanisms, including ion transport. The TEP is thereby altered, and wound healing is impaired. Biofilm or infection in the wound bed further compromises this healing cascade.

By directly working to restore these altered TEPs, the use of electrostimulation (ES) devices has gained popularity as a safe and effective adjuvant option when it comes to wound healing. The devices supply a direct, alternating, or pulsed current through electrodes embedded within pads directly applied to the limb near or on the wound. These currents create chemoelectric gradients that alter gene expression and activate intracellular signaling cascades to induce cell division, migration, and proliferation.[15] Several clinical studies, RCTs, and case reports have demonstrated the clinical efficacy of ES in chronic wounds, including ischemic ulcers when patients are compliant with therapy.

In a prospective, randomized, single-blinded, sham-controlled clinical trial by Goldman and colleagues, ischemic wounds, defined as transcutaneous oxygen pressure ($TcPO_2$) less than 20 mm Hg, were treated for 14 weeks with either high-voltage, pulsed current or a sham device. The authors found that compared with the sham, the wounds treated with ES had a significant decrease in size ($P < .05$) as well as a substantial improvement in periwound microcirculation based on laser Doppler ($P < .01$) and $TcPO_2$ ($P < .05$) measurements.[16]

In 2022, a systematic review analyzed the effects of ES on DFUs using data from 5 RCTs, one prospective study, and one retrospective study and found that while all wounds healed faster with ES compared with SOC, only wounds with an ischemic cause had a statistically significant increase in healing rate.[17] Although notable, the authors were hesitant to make definitive conclusions owing to the degree of bias and low power in the included studies.

A single-center, open-label study evaluating the effect of neuromuscular stimulation on the common peroneal nerve in 8 patients with ischemic ulcers using an ES device (geko, FirstKind Ltd, High Wycombe, UK) showed significantly increased flux and pulsatility in the wound beds and wound edges of all patients, indicating improved microvascular blood flow from ES in patients with ischemic wounds (**Fig. 2**).[18]

In early 2023, results from a randomized, double-blinded control study were published that further provided evidence to support the use of electrical stimulation in CLTI. In the study, 33 patients with chronic DFUs and mild-to-moderate PAD were randomized to undergo daily sessions with an ES device (Tennant Biomodulator PRO) or an identical, nonfunctional device for 4 weeks and found that wound area reduced by 22% ($P = .002$) in the treatment group. The control group had no significant change in wound area ($P = .982$).[19]

Oxygen therapy

Oxygen therapy aims to facilitate wound healing by increasing local oxygen levels within a poorly perfused wound bed. Hyperbaric oxygen therapy (HBOT), the more traditional approach, has well-recognized efficacy in chronic wound management, and its lesser-known counterpart, topical oxygen therapy (TOT), has begun to emerge

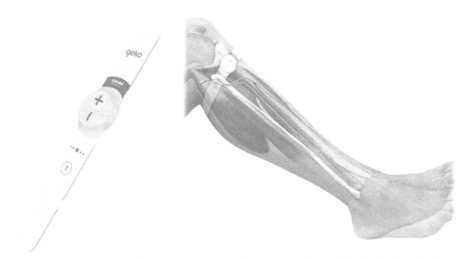

Fig. 2. The geko device. (Geko™ Device. With permission from Sky Medical Technology: https://www.gekodevices.com/.)

as possibly even more effective. Regardless, HBOT and TOT are uniquely distinct and clinically effective adjuncts for managing a range of ulcer etiologies, including ALUs.[20]

Hyperbaric oxygen therapy. HBOT is indicated as a primary therapy for a variety of acute conditions, including decompression sickness, carbon monoxide poisoning, air and gas embolisms, compartment syndrome, and acute arterial insufficiency.[21] As an adjunct, HBOT has been used for decades in treating chronic wounds. The therapeutic success of HBOT is based on the effect of inhaling high concentrations of oxygen. Placing a patient into a pressurized chamber 3 times higher than atmospheric pressure and administering 100% O_2 increases the oxygen concentration in plasma and the diffusion distance exponentially. With this exponential increase, a significantly higher oxygen concentration reaches ischemic tissue, which promotes neovascularization and is bacteriostatic and bactericidal. Furthermore, as demonstrated by its therapeutic efficacy in acute ischemia and reperfusion injuries, HBOT decreases the release of proteases and free radicals, which can decrease vasoconstriction, cell damage, and tissue swelling.[22]

Regarding clinical evidence supporting HBOT in ALUs, RCTs, let alone studies, are lacking. Most publications have focused on DFUs, and conclusions have been inconsistent due to flawed study designs, poor reporting, and low power.

However, in 2020, a meta-analysis by Laleiu and colleagues shed much-needed light on a critical factor that had yet to be fully addressed in earlier studies. The authors theorized that the inconsistencies in prior publications were actually due to a lack of distinction between patients with DFUs who had concurrent PAD and those who had DFUs of purely nonischemic cause. Based on a stratified analysis, they found that HBOT did not improve healing or amputation rate in patients with wounds of purely diabetic origin but may have some effect on patients with ulcers and PAD.[23]

Based on available clinical evidence, HBOT may have greater benefits than previously imagined in patients with both ischemic and nonischemic ulcers. However, larger power, double-blinded, and risk-stratified RCTs will be integral for better understanding. Nevertheless, in the patient with CLTI with no revascularization options, HBOT is a worthwhile option considering its widespread insurance coverage and minimal adverse effects. However, HBOT requires travel to a specific center, and therapy mandates frequent sessions for weeks at a time, so in some octogenarians, this may prove too cumbersome of an endeavor.

Topical oxygen therapy. TOT devices were initially introduced as a more convenient, lower cost alternative to HBOT without the associated adverse effects. By delivering low-pressurized oxygen from a chamber connected to a bag or boot, targeted oxygen is delivered directly to the affected limb or wound through diffusion, avoiding the risk of barotrauma, pneumothorax, or hypoglycemia, as reported with HBOT.[24]

Although original TOT devices were large, noisy, and constraining, requiring wall power and dedicated therapy sessions, newer TOT devices have come to market during recent years that are small, use disposable or rechargeable batteries, and can be worn by patients in an ambulatory setting. Some devices provide continuous oxygen or pressure, whereas others use cyclical pressurized and humidified oxygen.[24,25] Specialized dressings and oxygen emulsions have also been incorporated into therapy and have had varying clinical successes.[26]

Most clinical evidence supporting TOT has come from DFU studies but a handful of studies have also demonstrated efficacy in venous leg ulcers (VLUs), pressure ulcers (PUs), and ALUs. Unfortunately, due to low power, poor randomization, and insufficient blinding in these studies, TOT has not been widely incorporated into a standardized ischemic wound care algorithm.[24] Regardless, TOT remains a promising adjunct for healing chronic wounds.

Among the more notable DFU trials, an observational clinical trial (OTONAL) using a TOT device (Natrox® O_2, Inotec AMD., Cambridge, England) in patients with nonhealing DFUs, 90% of which had undergone revascularization for CLTI before TOT (**Fig. 3**), showed that after 3 months of TOT, 70% of patients had greater than 75% wound closure with a 91.3% wound area reduction ($P = .001$), and a significant decrease in pain scores ($P = .008$).[27]

In clinical practice, the efficacy of TOT for healing chronic VLUs and ALUs has also been favorable. In a small study by Kaufman and colleagues, TOT was prescribed to patients with chronic VLUs and ALUs in a tertiary care setting, and although only 32% of all wounds closed, after 25 days of TOT, ALU size decreased by 74% and 57% of ALUs closed.[28]

During recent years, a handful of studies assessing the role of TOT for ALUs in patients with revascularizable and nonrevascularizable anatomy have come to light, and findings have been favorable. In one single-center study by Valakh and colleagues, 28 patients with PAD and nonhealing ulcers underwent TOT 4 times a week after either

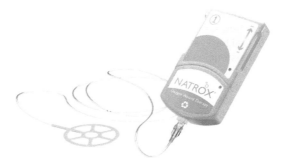

Fig. 3. NATROX® O_2 device. (NATROX® O2 Device. With permission from Inotec AMD Limited: https://www.natroxwoundcare.com/natrox-o2/.)

revascularization or debridement if the patient was not a revascularization candidate. After a maximum of 7 months of TOT, 25% of patients healed completely, and 66% had a reduction in wound area.[29]

A pilot study published in June 2023 further highlighted the improved efficacy of TOT when used as part of a multimodal treatment plan compared with SOC in patients with ALUs. In the study, 30 patients with nonhealing, ischemic ulcers were treated with either TOT combined with a specialized, silver-impregnated dressing or with the dressing alone. At 4 weeks, although both groups had statistically significant reductions in ulcer surface area, the percentage change in ulcer area in the treatment arm was much greater than in the control ($34.6 \pm 8.47\%$ vs $25.23 \pm 6.01\%$; $P = .003$). Decreased pain intensity was also significant in the TOT group compared with the control ($P = .002$).[30]

Although larger powered, unbiased RCTs are needed, the benefit of TOT as an adjunctive therapy for ischemic wounds is clear.

Stem cell therapy

Stem cell-based therapies have much potential in patients with chronic wounds owing to the intrinsic ability of stem cells to induce cell differentiation, proliferation, and migration through cytokine and growth factor upregulation, as well as promote neovascularization, collagen deposition, and epithelialization.[31] Following the therapeutic angiogenesis by cell transplantation (TACT) trial in 2002, which found an increased transcutaneous oxygen pressure ($TcPO_2$), ankle brachial index (ABI), and peak walking distance after intramuscular injection of bone marrow-derived mononuclear cells (BM-MNCs) compared with intramuscular injection of peripheral blood stem cells in patients with CLI, several small phase I and II RCTs were performed to explore these cell-based therapies.[32]

Although initial results from these smaller RCTs were initially promising, findings from larger, better-designed studies trials and placebo and meta-analyses failed to find significant differences in amputation rate and mortality. Nevertheless, considering the paucity of noninterventional options available for patients with CLTI and the numerous possibilities if harnessed effectively, research continued with autologous cell therapy but gears shifted toward new cell sources. Mesenchymal stem cells (MSCs), particularly, are of significant interest owing to their pluripotent nature and immunomodulatory and antibacterial properties that aid in regeneration and repair.[33]

A Cochrane review published in 2018 pooled data from 7 RCTs to compare the efficacy and safety of autologous cells from different sources, administered at different doses and given via different routes for "no-option" patients with CLTI. Studies compared BM-MNCs to peripheral blood stem cells, BM-MNCs to BM-MSCs, high and low doses, and intramuscular or intra-arterial administration routes. No difference was noted in amputation rate, rest pain scores, or TcO_2 among the studies; however, patients treated with BM-MSCs had a significantly greater number of healed ulcers, increased ABIs, and improved TcO_2 than those treated with BM-MNCs.[34]

MSCs sourced from the placenta have also demonstrated efficacy in ischemic wounds in several preclinical studies and clinical trials. Pluristem Therapeutics has completed a multinational placebo-controlled, parallel-group phase III trial (PACE Study) to evaluate the efficacy, tolerability, and safety of intramuscular injections of placenta-derived, allogenic, mesenchymal-like stromal cells (PLX-PAD) in "no-option" patients with CLTI with the primary endpoint of time to major amputation or death. Results from the study are currently still pending publication.[35] Furthermore, a single-arm, multicenter phase III trial has published promising results using off-the-shelf BM-MSCs (Stempeucel, Stempeutics, Bangalore, India) in 24 patients with CLI, showing significant improvements in rest pain and ulcer size, as well as increased ABI.[36]

Autologous cell therapy is an exciting therapeutic modality for no-option patients with CLTI, which holds much potential in the octogenarian for improving QOL, ischemic ulcer healing, and amputation-free survival. However, regardless of study size, randomization, or design, all study endpoints in all RCTs have consistently lost significance when placebo controls have come into play.

ARTERIAL REVASCULARIZATION OPTIONS AND OUTCOMES

Revascularization in the octogenarian represents a convergence of the multifaceted challenges inherent in geriatric medicine and vascular surgery. The pathophysiology underlying and potentiating ALUs is complex, involving a combination of macrovascular disease and microvascular issues that affect healing, such as endothelial dysfunction, prolonged inflammation, and impaired angiogenesis.[37] These factors are exacerbated by the physiologic changes of aging, including reduced vascular compliance, decreased responsiveness to nitric oxide, and increased propensity for thrombogenic activity.[38]

Open Surgery

Open surgical interventions include endarterectomy and arterial bypass, which can be performed separately or in tandem in one or multiple arterial segments to restore flow.

In the octogenarian, open revascularization can be challenging because age is an independent risk factor for adverse events, and functional reserve, the ability to endure the stress of surgery, and tissue healing are all affected by aging. Certain comorbidities, including coronary artery and cerebrovascular disease, diabetes, and chronic kidney disease, are more prevalent in this population and increase the risk for not only perioperative complications but also postoperative myocardial infarction, stroke, and infection.[39] Further, geriatric patients are particularly prone to developing postoperative delirium, which can at best, significantly lengthen hospital stay, and at worst, result in permanent disability and death.[40]

Surgical outcomes in this demographic are mixed. Age has been noted to be an independent predictor of acute graft failure and readmission in patients aged older than 80 years, and 30-day mortality postbypass is as high as 25.6% in octogenarians compared with 7.9% in those younger than 80 years after bypass in octogenarians compared with nonoctogenarians have been quoted as high as 25.6% versus 7.9% ($P < .001$), respectively.[41,42]

However, graft patency is comparable in octogenarians and younger cohorts with a 3-year patency exceeding 70%.[43] A recent study further showed that in octogenarians who underwent the same preoperative risk assessment as younger patients, there were no differences in primary patency, hospital stay, and limb salvage when all comorbidities were considered.[44]

Therefore, although limb salvage rates are high after the open intervention, the morbidity associated with complications can significantly affect the functional status and QOL, as well as increase mortality. The decision to proceed with surgery must be carefully weighed based on a patient's comorbidities. A clear discussion with the patient and caregivers regarding realistic expectations and potential outcomes is essential.

Endovascular Revascularization

Endovascular revascularization (EVR) with percutaneous angioplasty and stenting, when indicated, offers a minimally invasive alternative to open surgery for the octogenarian with a non-healing ALU (**Fig. 4**). EVR is associated with a lower rate of peri-interventional and postinterventional complications and shorter hospital stays than

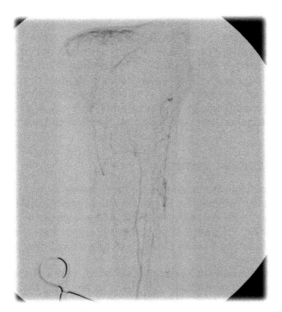

Fig. 4. Multivessel disease on angiogram.

open surgery, making it an attractive option for high-risk surgical patients.[45] However, EVR is not without complication, and dissections, perforations, distal embolization, bleeding, and contrast-induced kidney injury are all concerns.[46] Additionally, heavily calcified and tortuous vessels can increase the risk of complications and prohibit successful intervention.

Short-term patency in octogenarians after EVR has consistently been reported as equivalent to open surgery.[47] However, regarding long-term outcomes, EVR has been associated with markedly low primary and secondary patency, and reintervention rates are much higher than with open bypass.[48]

Therefore, EVR has a significant role in the comorbid octogenarian with an ALU but routine imaging surveillance to assess patency and medical therapy for optimization is paramount. Notably, the use of statins, antiplatelet agents, and, in some cases, anticoagulation has been independently associated with an improved survival in octogenarians after EVR.[49]

Hybrid Approaches

The combined use of endovascular intervention and surgical endarterectomy in patients with multilevel disease has increased in popularity during recent years for patients with ALUs with multilevel arterial occlusive disease. Compared with surgical bypass alone, complication and mortality rates have been reported as significantly lower when using a hybrid technique, and long-term patency has been considerably higher than in patients who underwent EVR alone.[48] In patients with CLTI, hybrid approaches have demonstrated particular efficacy for iliofemoral disease, wherein iliac stenting is performed with femoral endarterectomy. In a case series published by Kavanagh and colleagues, using this hybrid approach resulted in such significant increases in inflow that outflow revascularization became unnecessary in several patients.[50] However, its role in specifically the octogenarian population has not been formally evaluated, and clinical evidence has not been age-specific.

Venous Arterialization

During the last 2 decades, distal venous arterialization (DVA) has emerged as a viable last-resort option for patients with CLTI who are not candidates for open or EVR. By connecting a distal artery and vein via an open or percutaneous approach, arterial flow can be diverted into the distal tibial or plantar venous system to perfuse the distal lower limb. However, frequent surveillance and close follow-ups, lifestyle modifications, and adherence to medical therapies may prove difficult in some octogenarians, so the appropriateness of DVA must be evaluated case-by-case.

THE IMPACT OF FUNCTIONAL STATUS

The functional status of an octogenarian is a critical determinant of prognosis following arterial revascularization. Mobility, strength, cognition, and the ability to perform activities of daily living must all be considered. Preoperative assessment tools, such as the Barthel Index, the Short Physical Performance Battery, or the Frailty Scale, can provide a quantifiable measure to help stratify risk and inform discussions before proceeding with intervention.[51]

Frailty itself is associated with longer hospital stays, delirium, decline in functional status, and increased risk of mortality.[52] In the octogenarian, a decreased functional status preoperatively portends to higher mortality, an increased likelihood of postoperative complications, and a slower or unsuccessful return to baseline functioning after revascularization. When compared with ambulatory patients, nonambulatory octogenarians will also have much higher rates of reintervention, which not only adds to increased morbidity and health-care costs but also places a physical and psychological burden on the patient.[53]

An estimated 45% of geriatric patients will have some degree of functional decline after surgery.[54] In addition, 30% of geriatric patients will fall victim to hospital-associated deconditioning due to prolonged bed rest and immobility.[55] In the previously ambulatory and optimized octogenarian, these declines can be transient but in those with additional comorbidities or reduced mobility at baseline, a deconditioned state can persist and increase the likelihood of future amputation and death.[54] Depression, particularly in those who experience a decline postoperatively, is also a concern because it can significantly impede recovery and rehabilitation efforts.

Therefore, early mobilization programs, physical therapy, and occupational therapy are crucial in the postoperative care plan. These interventions can help prevent complications such as deep vein thrombosis, pressure ulcers, pneumonia, and delirium, which are more prevalent in the geriatric population.[56] Enhanced recovery after surgery protocols have been adapted to align with vascular surgery needs, and early mobilization plays a pivotal role in the patient's recovery.[57]

The decision to proceed with arterial revascularization in the octogenarian mandates a comprehensive assessment and discussion on a case-by-case basis. It requires a multidisciplinary treatment approach to care. Life expectancy, goals of care, comorbidities, functional status, and disease location are all critical considerations, and discussing risks, benefits, and potential complications is essential to ensure that the chosen path aligns with a patient's health-care goals and expectations.

In high-risk patients with multiple comorbidities and a decreased functional status, an endovascular-first approach can improve QOL without posing an additional risk to morbidity and survival. However, in the ambulatory octogenarian who has well-optimized comorbidities, proceeding with surgical bypass will likely offer a greater long-term benefit.

Algorithm of Care for the Octogenarian with an Arterial Leg Ulcer

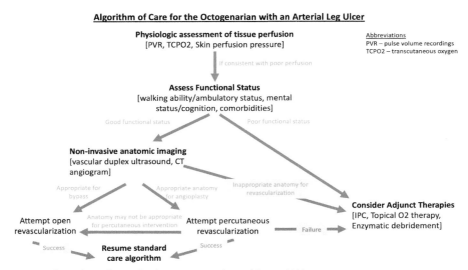

Fig. 5. Algorithm of care in the octogenarian with an ALU.

ALGORITHM FOR CARE

Without revascularization, an ALU will seldom heal, and in the nonrevascularizable octogenarian with CLTI, 30% will undergo major amputation, and 25% will die within 1 year.[5] Although the soon-to-be-published results from the PACE study may show that morbidity and mortality numbers continue to improve because of medical therapy, any attempt to restore flow must still be made in the octogenarian with an ALU if safe, appropriate, and reasonably achievable (**Fig. 5**).

Regarding the octogenarian who cannot undergo revascularization, we have succeeded in halting ALU progression, improving pain and QOL, and, in some cases, reducing ALU size by using a multimodal treatment algorithm that incorporates the TIME (Tissue debridement, Infection control, Moisture balance, and Edges of the wound) principles in conjunction with adjunctive therapies. We have found that permissive, enzymatic debridement using bacterial collagenase fermented from *Clostridium histolyticum* (SANTYL, Smith + Nephew, Watford, United Kingdom) coupled with TOT has been very effective.

Our institution has also found that specific cellular and tissue-engineered therapies have been promising in ALU healing. Specifically, acellular fish skin, powdered urinary bladder matrix, powdered porcine submucosa, and powdered amniotic tissues seem to generate granulation tissue in these ischemic wounds. Nevertheless, these therapies have only been studied in patients with nonischemic ulcers, so our recommendations are based solely on clinical practice observations.

SUMMARY

ALUs in the octogenarian population are complex, and their management requires a multifactorial approach that considers both macrovascular and microvascular disease. A wound care algorithm incorporating chronic wound management fundamentals is critical to successful outcomes after revascularization. In patients who are not candidates for intervention, these principles, coupled with TOT, HBOT, and IPC, have shown promise. Enhancing the QOL needs to be the focus of the intervention.

Additionally, using specific tissue therapies that tend to generate granulation tissue has proven effective at our institution. Although we recommend this multimodal algorithm when confronted with managing an ALU in a nonrevascularizable patient, there remains a lack of published clinical evidence to support our findings. Future studies that examine the role of cellular therapies in ischemic wounds and a better understanding of how microcirculation is affected and can be corrected in patients with ALUs will significantly benefit future care.

CLINICS CARE POINTS

- Revascularization remains the primary means of healing an arterial leg ulcer even in the octogenarian
- The elderly patients functional status, frailty, and goals of care must be considered when deciding on revascularization options
- Algorithms can augment or, even in some cases, replace revascularization to help patient has healed her lower extremity arterial wounds even when elderly

DISCLOSURE

A.L. Fierro, M Abeshouse, and T Lagziel have no commercial or financial conflicts of interest to disclose. J C. Lantis II has previously been an investigator for topical oxygen companies and currently serves as a consultant for Smith and Nephew, Organogenesis, Kerecis, and Integra. In addition, he is currently a principal investigator for MediWound, Organogenesis, and Biotissue. No grants nor payments from any company were received in regard to this academic study.

REFERENCES

1. Zemaitis MR, Boll JM, Dreyer MA. Peripheral arterial disease. Treasure Island (FL): StatPearls; 2023.
2. Criqui MH, Aboyans V. Epidemiology of peripheral artery disease. Circ Res 2015; 116(9):1509–26.
3. Moulik PK, Mtonga R, Gill GV. Amputation and mortality in new-onset diabetic foot ulcers stratified by etiology. Diabetes Care 2003;26(2):491–4.
4. Cutmore C, Aitken S. Managing chronic limb-threatening ischaemia in patients at the extremes of older age requires a patient-focused approach. World J Surg 2022;46(11):2832–3 [published Online First: 20220818].
5. Davies MG. Criticial limb ischemia: epidemiology. Methodist Debakey Cardiovasc J 2012;8(4):10–4.
6. Jude EB, Oyibo SO, Chalmers N, et al. Peripheral arterial disease in diabetic and nondiabetic patients: a comparison of severity and outcome. Diabetes Care 2001;24(8):1433–7.
7. Mayrovitz HN, Wong S, Mancuso C. Venous, arterial, and neuropathic leg ulcers with emphasis on the geriatric population. Cureus 2023;15(4):e38123.
8. Elkady R, Tawfick W, Hynes N, et al. Intermittent pneumatic compression for critical limb ischaemia. Cochrane Database Syst Rev 2018;2018(7):CD013072.
9. Kavros SJ, Delis KT, Turner NS, et al. Improving limb salvage in critical ischemia with intermittent pneumatic compression: a controlled study with 18-month follow-up. J Vasc Surg 2008;47(3):543–9.

10. Alvarez OM, Wendelken ME, Markowitz L, et al. Effect of high-pressure, intermittent pneumatic compression for the treatment of peripheral arterial disease and critical limb ischemia in patients without a surgical option. Wounds 2015;27(11):293–301.
11. Zaki M, Elsherif M, Tawfick W, et al. The role of sequential pneumatic compression in limb salvage in non-reconstructable critical limb ischemia. Eur J Vasc Endovasc Surg 2016;51(4):565–71.
12. Maan ZN, Januszyk M, Rennert RC, et al. Noncontact, low-frequency ultrasound therapy enhances neovascularization and wound healing in diabetic mice. Plast Reconstr Surg 2014;134(3):402e–11e.
13. Mohamad Yusoff F, Kajikawa M, Yamaji T, et al. Low-intensity pulsed ultrasound decreases major amputation in patients with critical limb ischemia: 5-year follow-up study. PLoS One 2021;16(8):e0256504.
14. Rajendran SB, Challen K, Wright KL, et al. Electrical stimulation to enhance wound healing. J Funct Biomater 2021;12(2). https://doi.org/10.3390/jfb12020040 [published Online First: 20210619].
15. Evans JP, Sen CK. Electrochemical devices in cutaneous wound healing. Bioengineering (Basel) 2023;10(6). https://doi.org/10.3390/bioengineering10060711 [published Online First: 20230611].
16. Goldman R, Rosen M, Brewley B, et al. Electrotherapy promotes healing and microcirculation of infrapopliteal ischemic wounds: a prospective pilot study. Adv Skin Wound Care 2004;17(6):284–94.
17. Melotto G, Tunprasert T, Forss JR. The effects of electrical stimulation on diabetic ulcers of foot and lower limb: a systematic review. Int Wound J 2022;19(7):1911–33.
18. Bosanquet DC, Ivins N, Jones N, et al. Microcirculatory flux and pulsatility in arterial leg ulcers is increased by intermittent neuromuscular electrostimulation of the common peroneal nerve. Ann Vasc Surg 2021;71:308–14.
19. Zulbaran-Rojas A, Park C, El-Refaei N, et al. Home-based electrical stimulation to accelerate wound healing-a double-blinded randomized control trial. J Diabetes Sci Technol 2023;17(1):15–24.
20. James CV, Park SY, Alabi D, et al. Effect of topical oxygen therapy on chronic wounds. Surg Technol Int 2021;39:51–7.
21. DuBose KJ, Cooper JS. Hyperbaric patient selection. Treasure Island (FL): StatPearls; 2023.
22. Jones MW, Cooper JS. Hyperbaric therapy for wound healing. Treasure Island (FL): StatPearls; 2023.
23. Lalieu RC, Brouwer RJ, Ubbink DT, et al. Hyperbaric oxygen therapy for nonischemic diabetic ulcers: a systematic review. Wound Repair Regen 2020;28(2):266–75 [published Online First: 20191126].
24. Patel M, Lantis JC 2nd. Management of non-reconstructable critical limb ischemia. Surg Technol Int 2019;34:69–75.
25. Oropallo A, Andersen CA. Topical oxygen. Treasure Island (FL): StatPearls; 2023.
26. Gold MH, Nestor MS. A supersaturated oxygen emulsion for wound care and skin rejuvenation. J Drugs Dermatol 2020;19(3):250–3.
27. Tang TY, Mak MYQ, Yap CJQ, et al. An observational clinical trial examining the effect of topical oxygen therapy (natrox) on the rates of healing of chronic diabetic foot ulcers (OTONAL Trial). Int J Low Extrem Wounds 2021. https://doi.org/10.1177/15347346211053694. 15347346211053694.
28. Kaufman H, Gurevich M, Tamir E, et al. Topical oxygen therapy stimulates healing in difficult, chronic wounds: a tertiary centre experience. J Wound Care 2018;27(7):426–33.

29. Vulakh GM, Hingorani AP, Ascher E, et al. Adjunctive topical oxygen therapy for wound healing in patients with peripheral arterial disease. Vascular 2023;31(4): 737–40.
30. Pasek J, Szajkowski S, Cieslar G. Application of topical hyperbaric oxygen therapy and medical active dressings in the treatment of arterial leg ulcers-a pilot study. Sensors (Basel) 2023;23(12). https://doi.org/10.3390/s23125582 [published Online First: 20230614].
31. Cooke JP, Meng S. Vascular regeneration in peripheral artery disease. Arterioscler Thromb Vasc Biol 2020;40(7):1627–34 [published Online First: 20200521].
32. Tateishi-Yuyama E, Matsubara H, Murohara T, et al. Therapeutic angiogenesis for patients with limb ischaemia by autologous transplantation of bone-marrow cells: a pilot study and a randomised controlled trial. Lancet 2002;360(9331):427–35.
33. Huerta CT, Voza FA, Ortiz YY, et al. Mesenchymal stem cell-based therapy for non-healing wounds due to chronic limb-threatening ischemia: a review of preclinical and clinical studies. Front Cardiovasc Med 2023;10:1113982 [published Online First: 20230201].
34. Abdul Wahid SF, Ismail NA, Wan Jamaludin WF, et al. Autologous cells derived from different sources and administered using different regimens for 'no-option' critical lower limb ischaemia patients. Cochrane Database Syst Rev 2018;8(8): CD010747 [published Online First: 20180829].
35. Norgren L, Weiss N, Nikol S, et al. PLX-PAD cell treatment of critical limb ischaemia: rationale and design of the PACE trial. Eur J Vasc Endovasc Surg 2019;57(4):538–45 [published Online First: 20190125].
36. Gupta PK, Shivashankar P, Rajkumar M, et al. Label extension, single-arm, phase III study shows efficacy and safety of stempeucel® in patients with critical limb ischemia due to atherosclerotic peripheral arterial disease. Stem Cell Res Ther 2023;14(1):60 [published Online First: 20230401].
37. Khalid KA, Nawi AFM, Zulkifli N, et al. Aging and wound healing of the skin: a review of clinical and pathophysiological hallmarks. Life (Basel) 2022;12(12). https://doi.org/10.3390/life12122142 [published Online First: 20221219].
38. Bachschmid MM, Schildknecht S, Matsui R, et al. Vascular aging: chronic oxidative stress and impairment of redox signaling—consequences for vascular homeostasis and disease. Ann Med 2013;45(1):17–36.
39. Jin F, Chung F. Minimizing perioperative adverse events in the elderly. Br J Anaesth 2001;87(4):608–24. https://doi.org/10.1093/bja/87.4.608.
40. Saarinen E, Vuorisalo S, Kauhanen P, et al. The benefit of revascularization in nonagenarians with lower limb ischemia is limited by high mortality. Eur J Vasc Endovasc Surg 2015;49(4):420–5. https://doi.org/10.1016/j.ejvs.2014.12.027.
41. Komshian SR, Lu K, Pike SL, et al. Infrainguinal open reconstruction: a review of surgical considerations and expected outcomes. Vasc Health Risk Manag 2017; 13:161–8 [published Online First: 20170508].
42. Kim Y, Cho BS, DeCarlo C, et al. Outcomes after femoropopliteal bypass in octogenarians. J Vasc Surg 2022;75(6):e198.
43. Hamdi A, Al-Zubeidy B, Obirieze A, et al. Lower extremity arterial reconstruction in octogenarians and older. Ann Vasc Surg 2016;34:171–7 [published Online First: 20160510].
44. Myers R, Mushtaq B, Taylor N, et al. Limb salvage in octogenarians with critical limb ischemia after lower extremity bypass surgery. J Vasc Surg 2023;78(1): 217–22. https://doi.org/10.1016/j.jvs.2023.02.022.
45. Shu H, Xiong X, Chen X, et al. Endovascular revascularization vs. open surgical revascularization for patients with lower extremity artery disease: a systematic

review and meta-analysis. Front Cardiovasc Med 2023;10:1223841 [published Online First: 20230724].

46. Thukkani AK, Kinlay S. Endovascular intervention for peripheral artery disease. Circ Res 2015;116(9):1599–613.

47. Huang HL, Jimmy Juang JM, Chou HH, et al. Immediate results and long-term cardiovascular outcomes of endovascular therapy in octogenarians and nonoctogenarians with peripheral arterial diseases. Clin Interv Aging 2016;11:535–43 [published Online First: 20160504].

48. Mustapha JA, Anose BM, Martinsen BJ, et al. Lower extremity revascularization via endovascular and surgical approaches: a systematic review with emphasis on combined inflow and outflow revascularization. SAGE Open Med 2020;8. https://doi.org/10.1177/2050312120929239. 2050312120929239.

49. Lakomek A, Köppe J, Barenbrock H, et al. Outcome in octogenarian patients with lower extremity artery disease after endovascular revascularisation: a retrospective single-centre cohort study using in-patient data. BMJ Open 2022;12(8): e057630 [published Online First: 20220801].

50. Kavanagh CM, Heidenreich MJ, Albright JJ, et al. Hybrid external iliac selective endarterectomy surgical technique and outcomes. J Vasc Surg 2016;64(5): 1327–34 [published Online First: 20160729].

51. Houghton JSM, Nduwayo S, Nickinson ATO, et al. Leg ischaemia management collaboration (LIMb): study protocol for a prospective cohort study at a single UK centre. BMJ Open 2019;9(9):e031257.

52. Kwak MJ. Delirium in frail older adults. Ann Geriatr Med Res 2021;25(3):150–9 [published Online First: 20210830].

53. Flu HC, Lardenoye JHP, Veen EJ, et al. Functional status as a prognostic factor for primary revascularization for critical limb ischemia. J Vasc Surg 2010;51(2): 360–71, e1.

54. Kwon S, Symons R, Yukawa M, et al. Evaluating the association of preoperative functional status and postoperative functional decline in older patients undergoing major surgery. Am Surg 2012;78(12):1336–44.

55. Loyd C, Markland AD, Zhang Y, et al. Prevalence of hospital-associated disability in older adults: a meta-analysis. J Am Med Dir Assoc 2020;21(4):455–61.

56. Aprisunadi Nursalam N, Mustikasari M, Ifadah E, et al. Effect of early mobilization on hip and lower extremity postoperative: a literature review. SAGE Open Nurs 2023;9. https://doi.org/10.1177/23779608231167825. 23779608231167825.

57. Stojanovic MD, Markovic DZ, Vukovic AZ, et al. Enhanced recovery after vascular surgery. Front Med 2018;5:2 [published Online First: 20180119].

Venous Leg Ulcers

The Need to Incorporate Age-Friendly 4M's in Management

Sarwat Jabeen, MD[a],[*], Elizabeth Foy White Chu, MD, CWSP, AGSF[b],[c]

KEYWORDS

- Venous reflux • Venous ulcer • Compression therapy

KEY POINTS

- Venous leg ulcer (VLU) accounts for 60% to 80% of the lower leg ulcers and more common in geriatric population.
- VLU entails complex underlying pathophysiology and several predisposing factors.
- Compression along with treating underlying predisposing factors is the key elements of management.
- Despite compression treatment and surgical and endovascular venous treatments, the overall healing and recurrence rate for VLU can be as high as 70%.

INTRODUCTION

It has been estimated that approximately 2.5 million people experience chronic venous insufficiency (CVI) in the United States, and of those about 20% develop venous leg ulcers (VLUs).[1] VLUs are the most common presentation of lower extremity wounds—as high as 80%.[2] As defined by the Society of Vascular Surgery and the American Venous Forum, a VLU is "an open skin lesion that occurs in an area affected by venous hypertension."[3] These seemingly innocuous lesions have a problematic high recurrence rate upward of 70% in 6 months.[4] Epidemiologic studies have demonstrated increasing prevalence with age, suggesting that VLUs are another wound-related geriatric syndrome.[5],[6]

The financial burden of VLUs is considerable. Medicare spending for this condition was $569 million in 2014 and ulcers that were infected added $146.7 million.[7] There is a loss of 4.6 million work-days per year.[8] With an aging population that seeks to

[a] Department of Family Medicine, Memorial Hermann Family Medicine Residency Program, 14023 Southwest Fwy, Sugar Land, TX 77478, USA; [b] Department of Geriatrics, Oregon Health & Science University, Portland VA Health Care System, 3710 SW US Veterans Hosp Road, Portland, OR 97239, USA; [c] Department of Medicine, Oregon Health and Sciences University, Wound Healing Service, Portland VA Health Care System, Portland, Oregon, USA
* Corresponding author. Michael E. DeBakey Department of Veterans Affairs, Room 2c-110, 2002 Holcombe Boulevard, Houston, TX 77030, USA
E-mail address: sarwat.jabeen@va.gov

Clin Geriatr Med 40 (2024) 413–436
https://doi.org/10.1016/j.cger.2023.12.009
0749-0690/24/© 2023 Elsevier Inc. All rights reserved.

geriatric.theclinics.com

continue employment either for necessity or pleasure, this has quality of life implications.

4 M'S IN THE CARE OF VENOUS LEG ULCERS

As referenced in the chapter "The Challenge of Chronic Wounds in Older Adults," we recommend that the clinician approach the VLU assessment with the 4M's in mind—what Matters Most, Medication, Mentation, and Mobility.[9] Wound closure should not be the presumed goal, especially for those patients who have lived with waxing/waning chronicity of this highly recurrent wound.

What Matters: The clinician will best serve the patient by asking them about their daily activities, what they enjoy doing most, and how the leg ulcers impair or prevent those activities altogether. A treatment plan can then be formed around this line of questioning.

Mobility: Immobility is a well-known risk factor for venous disease. The loss of the calf pump muscle function coupled with prolonged sitting in frail older adults can lead to vein dilation, skin changes, and possibly skin ulceration.[10] For those frail older adults with severe debility from dementia, spinal stenosis, or osteoarthritis, they may find it challenging to start an exercise program. Inquiring as to the cause of the immobility, the motivation for the patient to change and resources that are available are important endeavors in the treatment planning.

Medication: Although there are medications, such as pentoxifylline, that come with strong recommendations for use with compression therapy, the clinician must weigh the risk/benefits with polypharmacy. Polypharmacy is rampant among older adults; medication debridement should be the goal. There are some novel topical therapies, such as topical beta-blockers[11] and cannabis-based medications,[12] that if proven to be effective may serve our older adults better.

Compression wrapping is also the gold standard for VLU treatment and has been demonstrated to be so over years of investigative studies.[13] Compression wrapping is a medication—it requires a prescription as well as a clinician who has met competencies in applying it correctly. It is not without its complications.[14] A trained caregiver, licensed practical nurse (LPN) or registered nurse (RN), applies the wrapping two to three times per week, depending on the amount of drainage.

Mentation/Mood: Like many chronic diseases, prevention and treatment of VLUs requires diligence on the part of the patient and caregiver to minimize recurrence. This diligence is rooted in adequate daily hygiene to prevent cellulitis, mobility to don/doff garments, daily use of an intermittent pneumatic pressure device, daily aerobic programs, and daily calf raise exercises. When a VLU occurs, the patient needs transportation to and from wound clinics for advanced treatment planning and if they are homebound, access to home health aid (HHA) for two to three times a week compression wrapping. Like garments, there are considerable financial barriers to compression dressings.

One can imagine that the challenges those with cognitive impairment or dementia might face when having to stay on top of these daily tasks. The refrain of "I don't know why this is happening again" when they present to the clinic with a recurrence might very well lie in the patient's inability to remember to care for their legs and wear their garments. Clinicians need to have a low threshold to screen for cognitive disorders and address as best as possible in these patients.

DIAGNOSIS

In addition to history and physical examination, special consideration should be paid toward the causes of leg edema. Most likely the older adult with a swollen leg and ulcer will be due to venous insufficiency; there are other possibilities in the differential diagnosis (**Table 1**). Progression of venous insufficiency to the venous ulcer starts with the process of venous hypertension. Edema results from inadequate calf pump muscle function combined with venous obstruction or leakage. At the microlevel, there are breaks in capillary endothelium. This causes accumulation of inflammatory cells, which leads to obliteration of capillaries and resultant backflow pressure.

The CEAP classification (clinical, etiology, anatomy, and pathophysiology) has been developed to guide decision-making in CVI evaluation and treatment. The system has been shown to predict the patient's quality of life and the severity of their symptoms.[15] The CEAP classification is not always used by clinicians as by the time of diagnosis of the venous ulcer, the classification is C6. Higher scores than C6 do correlate with higher risk of developing leg ulcers and for ulcer recurrence. Someone who has had a leg ulcer is that much higher risk of developing a leg ulcer again. **Table 2** outlines common clinical findings in patients presenting with venous disease and VLUs.

Stasis dermatitis (SD) is a common result of venous insufficiency with venous hypertension. On clinical examination, SD appears as scaly, poorly demarcated, erythematous patches and plaques. The medial malleolar area is frequently and severely involved. The lower third of leg "gaiter area" is most involved but may extend down to the feet or up to the knees.

Significant reflux in external iliac vein, common femoral, vein, and saphenofemoral junction should raise suspicion for central venous pathology, especially on the left side. An underdiagnosed condition, May–Thurner syndrome, is this variant (**Fig. 1**). This condition is present in 20% of the population.[16] Compression of the left common iliac vein by the right common iliac artery in the pelvis causes an acute left iliofemoral deep vein thrombosis (DVT) or chronic left lower extremity edema. Consider this diagnosis in patients with recurrent DVT and unilateral left-side swelling. Management requires angioplasty with at least 6 months of anticoagulation.

VASCULAR ASSESSMENT

The Society for Vascular Surgery and Venous Leg Forum recommends that a comprehensive venous duplex ultrasound be performed if VLU is suspected.[3] Venous duplex is the only noninvasive test to check both patency and valvular competency of the deep, superficial, and perforator system. This test provides a roadmap of the venous anatomy as well as hemodynamic information about obstruction, valvular dysfunction, and venous reflux.[17] Patency of the vein and competency of the venous valve can affect the iliofemoral region, the superficial venous system, the deep venous system, or even the perforators. In true VLUs, there is usually an associated incompetent perforator.[17–19] If there is obstruction from previous ileofemoral venous thrombosis, the obstruction can potentially be treated with venous angioplasty and stenting. This procedure may improve edema and help heal ulcers as well as prevent recidivism.

Additional confirmatory diagnostic testing may include venography, plethysmography, ambulatory venous pressure measurement, radiography, and computed tomography.[17,19] Decision to order any of these tests should be done in collaboration with a vascular specialist.

Arterial examination and measurement of ankle brachial index (ABI) are recommended for all patients who are being managed for VLUs (**Table 3**). At times, it is difficult to palpate dorsalis pedis and posterior tibial with leg edema; a bedside handheld Doppler can be helpful but is subjective. If there are triphasic signals then this is reassuring. Biphasic or monophasic signals should push the provider for formal assessment. Ankle-brachial index and toe-brachial index are recommended. Older adult

Table 1
Differential diagnosis of venous leg ulcers

Type of Ulcer	Etiology	Location/Appearance	Management
Arterial ulcer	Tissue hypoxia due to atherosclerotic occlusions of leg arteries	Distal extremity like toes, foot lower legs Painful, punched out, deeper.	Based on the severity of arterial disease which is evaluated by ABI/TBI. Mild PAD can be managed by traditional wound care. Moderate to severe needs vascular consultation.

Mixed arterial
and venous

Combination of both venous and
    arterial disease

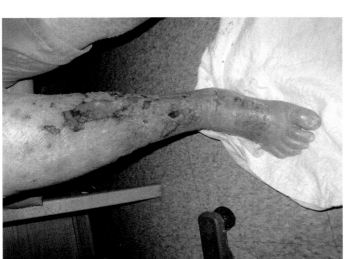

Treat possible cause of active ulcer
    based on appearance.
If ABI >0.5 and an absolute ankle
    pressure >60 mm Hg, compression
    up to 40 mm Hg does not impede
    arterial perfusion.

(continued on next page)

Table 1
(continued)

Type of Ulcer	Etiology	Location/Appearance	Management
Lymphatic ulcer	Phlebolymphedema	Shallow, lymphorrhea, positive Stemmer's sign	Lymphedema therapist Intermittent pneumatic compression device Specialized compression wrapping

| Martorell ulcer | Ischemic lesion of the tissue caused by obstruction of the small arterioles of the medial artery. | Punch biopsy for confirmation | Control of hypertension, preferred drugs calcium channel blocker, angiotensin-converting enzyme inhibitors (ACEI), pain control. Early skin graft shows better outcome |

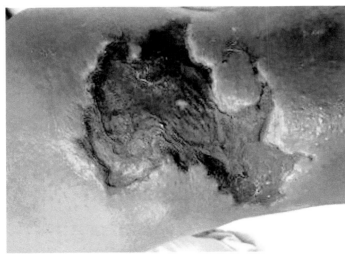

(continued on next page)

Table 1
(continued)

Type of Ulcer	Etiology	Location/Appearance	Management
Vasculitis ulcer	Injury of cutaneous microvessels leads to impairment of blood flow and consequent focal ischemia and formation of skin ulcers.	Ulcers are often multiple and located to lower legs. Very painful.	Traditional wound care and treatment of underlying disease, for example, autoimmune disease, drugs

| Pyoderma gangrenosum | Rapid progression of a painful, necrolytic cutaneous ulcer with an irregular, violaceous, and undermined border. Pathergy phenomenon with cribriform scarring | Often located in lower extremities Punch biopsy carries risk of pathergy. Biopsy may show neutrophilic infiltration. Dermatopathologist necessary to do final read. Often nonspecific findings and is clinical diagnosis. | Stepwise approach for the treatment including topical steroid cream intralesional and may need high-dose oral prednisone and other immunosuppressives. Treatment of underlying diseases, for example, inflammatory bowel disease. Conservative sharp debridement only to remove necrotic tissue |

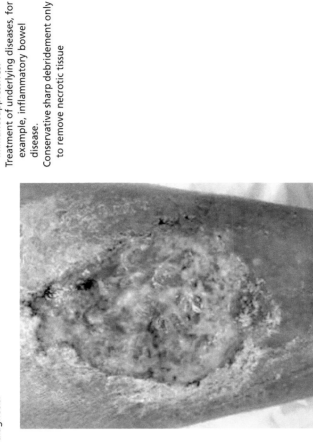

Abbreviations: ABI, ankle/brachial index; TBI, toe/brachial index; PAD, peripheral arterial disease.

Table 2
Common clinical findings in patients presenting with venous disease

Findings	Definition	Example
Varicose veins	Dilated superficial veins	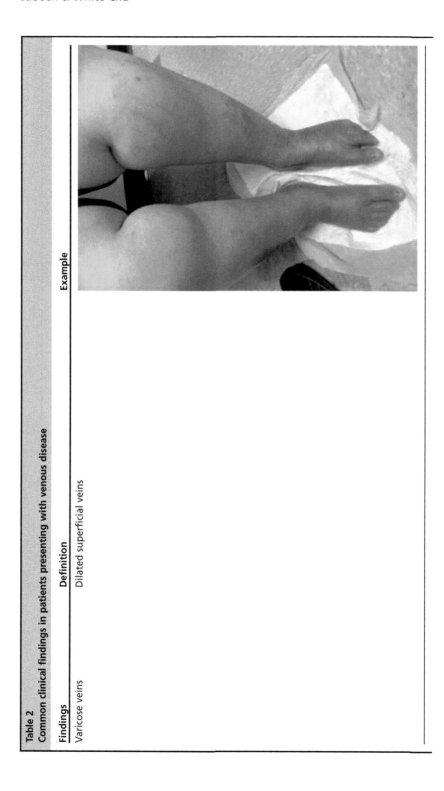

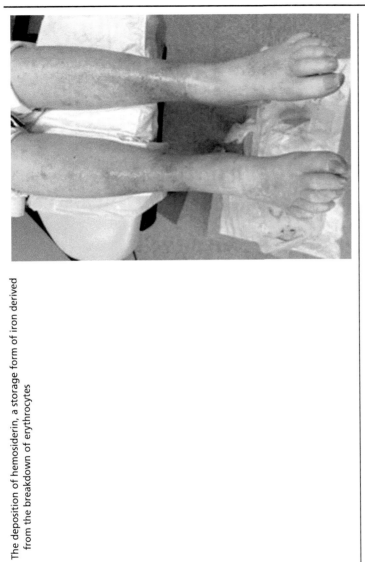

(continued on next page)

Hemosiderosis

The deposition of hemosiderin, a storage form of iron derived from the breakdown of erythrocytes

Table 2
(continued)

Findings	Definition	Example
Atrophie blanche	Star-shaped or polyangular, ivory-white depressed atrophic plaques, seen after healed venous ulcer	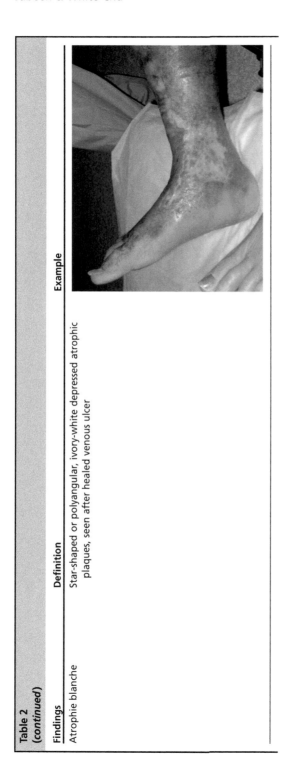

Corona phlebectatica /telangiectasia

Fan-shaped pattern of numerous small intradermal veins on either sides of ankle

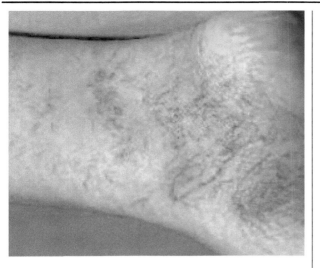

(continued on next page)

Table 2
(continued)

Findings	Definition	Example
Lipodermatosclerosis	Chronic inflammation, fat degeneration, and fibrosis	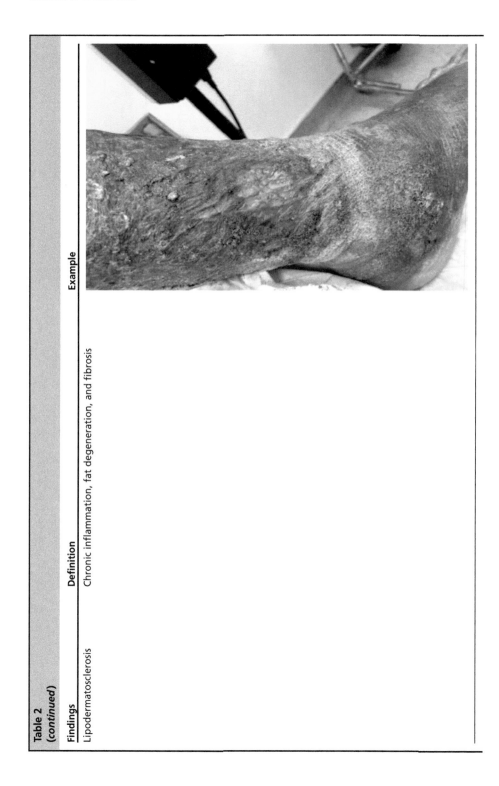

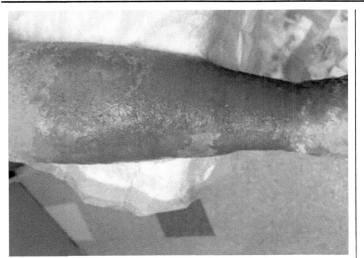

(continued on next page)

Stasis dermatitis

Inflammatory dermatosis of the lower extremities; often confused with cellulitis and can lead to cellulitis

Table 2
(continued)

Findings	Definition	Example
Nostras verrucosa	Chronic phlebolymphedema that causes progressive cutaneous hypertrophy	

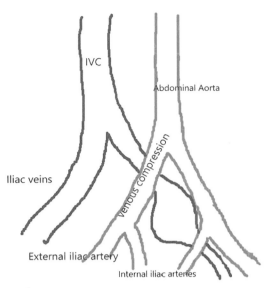

IVC

Abdominal Aorta

Iliac veins

venous compression

External iliac artery

Internal iliac arteries

Fig. 1. May–Thurner sydrome.

values may be falsely elevated due to calcification of the vessel wall and hardening of the medial layer. For those ulcers with mixed venous and arterial disease, it is vital to know the extent of the arterial disease severity. Compression is the key treatment for VLUs and must be done safely and competently. If the ABI is greater than 0.5 and absolute ankle pressure is greater than 60 mm Hg, then compression up to 40 mm Hg does not impede arterial perfusion.[20]

MANAGEMENT

When addressing VLU development, consider the underlying conditions that predispose the patient to leg edema and wounds. Common conditions include poorly controlled heart failure, renal failure, liver failure, and obstructive sleep apnea. Avoid compression therapy if there is acutely poor control of heart, renal, or liver failure. Chronic forms of these diseases do not contradict the need for compression. When determining how to address the ulcer, refer to infection/bioburden control, pain management, and wound bed preparation in other chapters of this publication.

- Compression therapy: Because venous ulcer development is sequela of venous reflux and venous hypertension, compression is the key. As mentioned earlier, before starting compression therapy, complete an arterial assessment to avoid arterial compromise. Compression increases venous return, improves muscle pump function, reduces edema from capillary leaks, improves lymphatic flow, and works against the chronic local inflammatory state that leads to poor healing and ulcer recurrence.[21]The delivery of compression comes in many forms (**Table 4**).[22] Compression bandages are available from a single bandage to multiple component bandages, including elastic, inelastic, or a combination. Major goals of compression therapy for VLUs are both ulcer healing and prevention of recurrence. Consider the patient's tolerance for compression wrap. An ideal wrap is cost-effective, comfortable, easy to apply and remove, and exerts therapeutic pressure. For wheelchair users patients who are unable to apply or

Table 3
Ankle brachial indices interpretations

Index	Signs and Symptoms	Disease Severity	Management
>0.7–1	Mild intermittent claudication or no symptoms	Mild arterial disease	Risk factors modification includes smoking cessation, graduated walking program, and weight loss. Consider referral to peripheral arterial disease rehabilitative program.
0.7–0.5	Intermittent claudication with variable severity	Mild to moderate arterial disease	In addition to above, referral to outpatient vascular specialist and possible arterial imaging (duplex scan or angiogram)
0.5–0.3	Severe intermittent claudication and rest pain	Severe arterial disease	In addition to above measures, urgent referral to vascular specialist and possible arterial imaging (duplex scan and/or angiogram)
<0.3	Critical ischemia (rest pain > 2 wk) with or without tissue loss (ulcer, gangrene)	Risk of limb loss	Vascular emergency, on call person needs to be contacted for possible surgical or radiological intervention

unable to tolerate compression bandaging, daily application of an intermittent pneumatic compression (IPC) for several hours stimulates blood flow and counteract edema. This can be used either in addition to or instead of compression bandaging.[23]

Non-Elastic Versus Elastic Bandages

The static stiffness index (SSI) is the difference between standing and resting pressure. Highly elastic products have an SSI of less than 10 mm Hg, whereas highly inelastic can be as high as greater than 50 mm Hg. Highly inelastic bandages remain stiff and resist geometric changes during activity, thus intermittently increasing pressure. This causes intermittent constricting of the veins, counteracting reflux and working against venous hypertension.[23]

Compression bandaging can be changed between 3 and 7 days depending on the drainage and how well the product resists sagging. Multicomponent wrapping often must be changed a minimum of twice weekly, whereas an Unna boot can stay in place for 7 days. Multicomponent systems are more effective than single-component systems, and two-component systems are as effective as four-layer systems.[22] There are repeated studies to support some compression over none for healing venous leg wounds.[13]

An Unna boot is a type of inelastic wrap that is an option for primary care doctors, given its cost and ease of use. This bandaging is impregnated with only zinc or a combination of zinc and calamine. It provides low compression (18–24 mm Hg). For this reason, an Unna boot can be used with mild to moderate peripheral arterial disease. Use with caution if ABI is between 0.5 and 0.8.[24] Avoid an Unna boot if there is sensitivity to zinc.

- Stasis Dermatitis: SD is the combination of venous hypertension and subcutaneous fluid accumulation. An influx of inflammatory cells in perivascular space leads to trophic skin changes and an eczematous skin condition. Distinguish acute SD from cellulitis to avoid exposure to unnecessary antibiotics.[25] If there

Table 4
Types of compressions for venous stasis ulcers and venous hypertension/leg edema

Compression Type	Examples	Level of Support	Mixed Arterial and Venous Disease	Mode of Action
Multicomponent: both elastic and inelastic components; two-layer non-inferior to four layers	Profore ($$) DynaFlex ($$) Velfour ($$) UrgoK2 ($$) Coban2 ($$)	High compression bandage system (SBP of 35–40 mm Hg at the ankle) Incorporates elastic layers to achieve sustained compression Layer 1: orthopedic wool Layer 2: cotton crepe bandage Layer 3: elastic compression bandage maintains SBP of 20 mm Hg at ankle Layer 4: cohesive compression bandage to retains the bandage in position and maintain a pressure of 30 mm Hg at the ankle	ABI 0.8–1.0 use high compression ABI 0.5–0.7 use light compression (layers 1, 2, and 4) ABI <0.5 or below: contraindicated, consult vascular team Provide equal pressure distribution. Requires competency apply it.	Reduces ambulatory venous pressure Increases venous refilling time Improves calf pump function
Inelastic	Unna boot ($) Cohesive bandage ($$) Velcro wraps: CircAid ($$$) ReadyWrap ($$$)	20–30 mm Hg 30–40 mm Hg As high as 40–50 mm Hg but depends on application	ABI 0.8–1.0 use high compression ABI 0.5–0.7 use light compression ABI <0.5 or below: contraindicated, consult vascular team Requires competency apply it.	Causes intermittent restriction of the veins during activity that prevents leaking of fluids to extravascular space. Better option for ambulatory patients.
Elastic	Ace wrap ($) Compression stockings ($) Tubular bandages ($)	ACE wrap with provides 14–17 mm Hg Higher compression provides 25–35 mm Hg	Avoid with obstructive arterial disease	Less working pressure, more resting pressure. ACE wrap has risk of quickly removing edema and then causing tourniquet on skin. Use with caution.

(continued on next page)

Table 4
(continued)

Compression Type	Examples	Level of Support	Mixed Arterial and Venous Disease	Mode of Action
Intermittent pneumatic compression (IPC)	Sequential compression therapy ($$$)	Varies, higher pressure around ankle than calf area	Can be used when concomitant arterial disease is detected	Increase flow velocity in the deep vein Increases local fibrinolysis, which decreases pericapillary cuffing Decreases interstitial edema by shifting fluid Improves arterial inflow by increasing the arteriovenous pressure gradient which causes release of endothelial derived relaxing factor Ideally done as 45 min treating in a bed or chair per day, thus restricting activity and potentially quality of life

is bilateral lower extremity erythema and edema, this condition is unlikely to be cellulitis.

SD that occurs in the setting of the tissue edema can be treated with topical steroids, regardless of the type of compression.[26] The bandaging alone will alleviate symptoms of inflammation, itching, and eczema.

- Mobilize: A systematic review and meta-analysis suggested that patients benefit from aerobic exercise with progressive resistance calf strengthening to improve ulcer healing. This comprehensive study noted that the evidence base has shifted in such a manner as to make this a standard recommendation.[27] Of those guidelines reviewed, only the clinical practice guidelines of the Society of Vascular Surgery (SVS) and American Venous Forum (AVF) acknowledge the importance of improving strength of the calf pump muscle. This guideline emphasizes the importance of self-management programs, structured exercise, and regular coaching and feedback.[3]
- Social Isolation: Patients with chronic VLUs suffer from physical, psychological, and social symptoms. Physically, there is odor, drainage, and leg swelling, which affect functional ability and physical appearance.[28] This can be psychologically exhausting to cope with dressing changes, manage expenses, and control co-morbidities. Patients my isolate themselves because of embarrassment or fatigue. Social isolation has damaging effects on health and contributes to the development of multiple chronic conditions and diminished healing.[29] Clinicians must screen patients for depression and isolation and address those conditions as part of a robust treatment plan.
- Additional Considerations: When a VLU finally closes, the guidelines are quite clear that a compression garment—such as stockings or velcro wrappings—must be prescribed and donned and doffed daily for the remainder of the older adult's life. The Society of Vascular Surgery on the Guideline of Invasive Treatment of Superficial Veins noted that there are challenges with donning/doffing stockings.[30] Like compression wrapping, the garments require technical ability on the part of the older adult to have strength and mobility in the hands and torso to pull on these stockings. Those with increased abdominal girth and/or arthritic conditions will find this task insurmountable, resulting in non-adherence to the garment. The guideline encourages the consideration of Velcro compression devices instead of stockings for these patients.

The efficacy of the newer, minimally-invasive endovenous techniques has been established in uncomplicated superficial venous disease, and these techniques can also be used in the management of VLU. When used with compression, endovenous ablation aims to further reduce pressure in the veins of the leg, which may impact ulcer healing.[31]

For chronic non-healing VLUs, pentoxifylline can be an effective adjunct. The guidelines provide a strong recommendation to use pentoxifylline with compression therapy for VLU management. Despite this recommendation, it is not common practice.[32] The medication must be taken three times per day, has significant gastrointestinal side effects, and interacts with antiplatelet medications. In the absence of compression, pentoxifylline also seems to be effective for treating edema.[33]

SUMMARY

Using the Age-Friendly System as a framework for the care of our older adults living with VLUs has potential to validate this geriatric syndrome and further support policy initiatives. For policymakers, the management needs to be geared toward the entire spectrum of care of VLU healing, especially for our frailest older adults. These patients need the most resources that include time intensive treatments, easy access to care, and prevention of immobilization. As national associations start to revise their VLU guidelines, they should consider how to integrate these nuances of geriatric medicine.

CLINICS CARE POINTS

- Venous Leg Ulcers are a common outcome of peripheral venous insufficiency and venous hypertension.
- 4M's of Geriatrics must be incorporated into venous leg ulcers as it is a Geriatric Syndrome.
- Management should address underlying issues of venous hypertension along with external compression if appropriate.
- Minimally invasive techniques help with ulcer healing for uncomplicated superficial venous disease.
- Address co-existing arterial disease with the help of vascular team.

DISCLOSURE

The authors have no financial affiliations or conflicts of interest.

REFERENCES

1. Rhodes JM, Gloviczki P, Canton LG, et al. Factors affecting clinical outcome following endoscopic perforator vein ablation. Am J Surg 1998;176:162–7.
2. O'Donnell TF, Balk EM. The need for an Intersociety Consensus Guideline for venous ulcer. J Vasc Surg 2011;54:83–90S.
3. O'Donnell, Passman MA, Marston WA, et al. Management of venous leg ulcers: clinical practice guidelines of the society for vascular Surgery® and the American venous Forum. J Vasc Surg 2014;60:3S–59S.
4. Gethen G, Killeen F, Devane D. Heterogenity of wound outcomes measures in RCTS of treatments for VLUs: a systematic review. J Wound Care 2015;24(5):211–2, 214, 216 passim.
5. Ruckley CV, Evans CJ, Allan PL, et al. Chronic venous insufficiency: clinical and duplex correlations. The Edinburgh Vein Study of venous disorders in the general population. J Vasc Surg 2002;36:520–5.
6. Margolis DJ, Bilker W, Santanna J, et al. Venous leg ulcer: incidence and prevalence in the elderly. J Am Acad Dermatol 2002;46:381–6.
7. Nussbaum SR, Carter MJ, Fife CE, et al. An economic evaluation of the impact, cost, and Medicare policy implications of chronic nonhealing wounds. Value Health 2018;21:27–32.
8. Spentzouris G, Labropoulos N. The evaluation of lower-extremity ulcers. Semin Intervent Radiol 2009;26(4):286–95.
9. Fulmer T, Pelton L, editors. Age-friendly systems: a guide to using the 4Ms while caring for older adults. Institute for Healthcare Improvement; 2022.
10. Abbade LPF, Lastoria S. Venous ulcer: epidemiology, physiopathology, diagnosis and treatment. The International Society of Dermatology 2005;44:449–56.

11. Baltazard T, Senet P, Momar D, et al. Evaluation of timolol maleate gel for management of hard-to-heal chronic venous leg ulcers. Phase II randomized-controlled study. Ann Dermatol Venereol 2021;148(4):228–32.
12. Maida V, Shi RB, Fazzari FGT, et al. Topical cannabis-based medicines – a novel adjuvant treatment for venous leg ulcers: an open-label trial. Exp Dermatol 2021; 30(9):1258–67.
13. Shi, Dumville JC, Cullum N, et al. Compression bandages or stockings versus no compression for treating venous leg ulcers. Cochrane Database Syst Rev 2021;7: CD013397.
14. Rabe E, Partsch H, Morrison N, et al. Risks and contraindications of medical compression treatment – a critical reappraisal. An international consensus statement. Phlebology 2020;35(7). 447-460.
15. Chamanga ET. Understanding venous leg ulcers. Br J Community Nurs 2018; 23(Sup9). S6-S15.
16. Peters M, Syed RK, Katz M, et al. May-Thurner syndrome: a not so uncommon cause of a common condition. SAVE Proc 2012;25(3):231–3. https://doi.org/10.1080/08998280.2012.119288.
17. Ren SY, Liu YS, Zhu GJ, et al. Strategies and challenges in the treatment of chronic venous leg ulcers. World J Clin Cases 2020;8(21):5070–85.
18. Raju S, Knepper J, May, et al. Ambulatory venous pressure, air plethysmography, and the role of calf venous pump in chronic venous disease. J Vasc Surg Venous Lymphat Disord 2019;7(3):428–40.
19. Krishnan S, Nicholls SC. Chronic venous insufficiency: clinical assessment and patient selection. Semin Intervent Radiol 2005;22(3):169–77.
20. Mosti G, Iabichella ML, Partsch H. Compression therapy in mixed ulcers increases venous output and arterial perfusion. J Vasc Surg 2012;55:122–8.
21. Nair B. Compression therapy for venous leg ulcers. Indian Dermatolo Online J 2014;5(3):378–82.
22. O'Meara S, Cullum N, Nelson EA, et al. Compression for venous leg ulcers. Cochrane Database Syst Rev 2012;11. Art No.: CD000265.
23. Partsch H. Intermittent pneumatic compression in immobile patients. Int Wound J 2008 Jun;5(3):389–97.
24. British Columbia Provincial Nursing Skin and wound committee (2016). Guideline: application of compression therapy to manage venous insufficiency and mixed venous/arterial insufficiency.
25. Hirschmann JV, Raugi GJ. Lower limb cellulitis and its mimics: part II. Conditions that simulate lower limb cellulitis. J Am Acad Dermatol 2012;67(2):177, e1-9; quiz 185-6.
26. Dissemond J, Knab J, Lehnen M, et al. Successful treatment of stasis dermatitis with topical tacrolimus. Vasa 2004;33(4):260–2.
27. Jull A, Slark J, Parsons J. Prescribed exercise with compression vs compression alone in treating patients with venous leg ulcers: a systematic review and meta-analysis. JAMA Dermatology 2018;154(11):1304–11.
28. Phillips P, Lumley E, Duncan R, et al. A systematic review of qualitative research into people's experiences of living with venous leg ulcers. J Adv Nurs 2018;74(3): 550–63.
29. Petitte T, Mallow J, Barnes E, et al. A systematic review of loneliness and common chronic physical conditions in adults. Open Psychol J 2015;8(Suppl 2):113–32.
30. Lurie, Lal BK, Antignani PL, et al. Compression therapy after invasive treatment of superficial veins of the lower extremities: clinical practice guidelines of the American venous Forum, society for vascular Surgery, American college of phlebology,

society for vascular medicine, and international union of phlebology. J Vasc Surg 2019;7(1):17–28.

31. Cai PL, Hitchman LH, Mohamed AH, et al. Endovenous ablation for venous leg ulcers. Cochrane Database Syst Rev 2023;7(7):CD009494.

32. Jull A, Walker N, Parag V, et al. Venous ulcer management in New Zealand: usual care versus guideline recommendations. NZ Med J 2009;122(1295):9–18.

33. Jull AB, Arroll B, Parag V, et al. Pentoxifylline for treating venous leg ulcers. Cochrane Database Syst Rev 2012;12(12):CD001733.

Diabetic Foot Ulcers in Geriatric Patients

Arthur Stone, DPM[a],*, Cornelius Michael Donohue, DPM, ACFAS[b]

KEYWORDS

- DFU • Diabetic ulcer • Plantar wounds • Wound healing

KEY POINTS

- Diabetic patients are prone to developing foot infections without the usual signs and symptoms such as redness, pain, and elevated white blood cell count.
- Care of DFU requires systematic communication with the PCP and other specialists to ensure optimal management of host factors necessary for healing.
- Patients should be educated on prevention, including foot care and lifestyle choices including smoking, drug and alcohol abuse.
- Many wounds require multiple debridements to maintain absence of necrotic tissue and resolve infection.
- Debrided tissue needs time to revascularize through angiogenesis, and edema needs time to reduce in preparation for primary closure or grafting.
- It is important to evaluate patients with a history of soft-tissue infection or osteomyelitis to assess for ongoing residual infection, including chronic refractory osteomyelitis (CRO).
- While most patients with DFUs heal within one year after receiving correct and adequate treatment, the recurrence rate remains high. Prevention of recurrence is an important aspect of management.

INTRODUCTION

This article will review pathophysiology, prevention, and management of diabetic foot ulcers (DFUs), both medical and surgical; and the importance of a systematic approach to diagnosis and treatment with emphasis on the team approach. In addition, global applications of the system of care will be discussed. The authors will review dermatologic, neurologic, metabolic, and immunologic aspects of DFU and impact of comorbidities such as obesity, hyperglycemia, and renal disease. Optimal outcomes can only be achieved by designing a personal Plan for Healing, including, rehabilitation, and prevention of recurrence. This begins with a thorough history and physical examination followed by differential diagnosis, appropriate laboratory,

[a] MedNexus, Inc., 1 Applewood Drive, Greenville, SC 29615, USA; [b] World Walk Foundation, 116 Whitemarsh Road, Ardmore, PA 19003, USA
* Corresponding author.
E-mail address: drartstone@bellsouth.net

Clin Geriatr Med 40 (2024) 437–447
https://doi.org/10.1016/j.cger.2024.03.002
0749-0690/24/© 2024 Elsevier Inc. All rights reserved.

radiologic, vascular and special studies, consultations and second opinions, and discussion with the patient, their families and/or Power of Attorney (POA).[1] Only after all these evaluations and communications are complete can a Plan for Healing be designed and implemented in order to obtain optimal outcomes.

Managing DFUs in geriatric patients creates additional challenges considering their medical and functional co-morbidities that will impact wound healing, including frailty and sarcopenia. However, the information and principles discussed in this article are applicable to diabetics of any age across the spectrum of diabetes types. As with all chronic wounds, prevention remains a key element of diabetic management.[2,3]

ACUTE AND CHRONIC WOUNDS

In healthy persons, an acute wound passes predictably through the phases of wound healing resulting in complete and sustained repair. Acute wounds typically occur in recently uninjured and otherwise normal tissue. The entire process is completed within 6 to 12 weeks, depending on the original depth of tissue involved.

Wounds that have not progressed through the normal process of healing and are unhealed for more than a month are classified as chronic wounds. There are multiple etiologies of chronic wounds, all of which burden the health care system. Patients suffering from diabetes and obesity are at a high risk of developing chronic wounds.Usually, the vast majority of people with chronic wounds also have other concomitant major health conditions.[4]

A central consideration regarding healing outcomes for DFUs and other types of wounds is the importance of early diagnosis, and initiation of early treatment.[5] This will optimize viable tissue maintenance and ambulatory function before further deterioration and infection occurs in soft-tissue and bone, which can lead to amputation and increased risk of mortality from sepsis. Principles discussed in this article apply to all acute and chronic wounds, regardless of etiology, including crush, laceration, puncture, abrasion, and thermal wounds.

EPIDEMIOLOGY OF DIABETIC FOOT ULCERS

A DFU is a debilitating, often recurrent, and severe manifestation of uncontrolled and prolonged diabetes that presents as ulceration, usually located on the plantar aspect of the foot (**Fig. 1**).[6] DFUs can occur on the lateral or medial aspects of the foot with varus and valgus structural and functional foot deformities, particularly if complicated

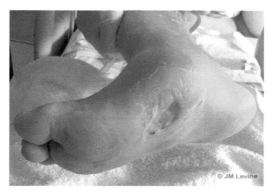

Fig. 1. Typical diabetic ulcer on plantar aspect of foot. (*Courtesy of* Jeffrey M. Levine, MD, AGSF, CMD.)

by digital and metatarsal deformities, and anatomic distortion related to diabetic Charcot neuro-arthropathy.[7] The pathologic mechanisms underlying DFUs comprise a triad, including neuropathy, vascular insufficiency, and secondary infection after trauma to the foot. Standard local and surgical care along with novel approaches like stem cell therapy, allo-, xeno-, and autografts, as well as off-loading strategies, pave the way to reduce morbidity, decrease amputations, and prevent disability from DFUs.[8]

Diabetes mellitus affects approximately 422 million people worldwide and is responsible for an estimated 2 million deaths per year.[9,10] It affects 11.3% of the United States population. Approximately 15% of individuals with diabetes will eventually develop 1 of these ulcers and, and out of these, 14% to 24% will require amputation of the ulcerated foot due to bone infection or other complications such as necrotizing fasciitis or limb ischemia. With a high level of morbidity stemming from osteomyelitis and amputation, it is of utmost importance to address and treat the underlying causes of DFU.

The International Diabetes Foundation estimates that 40 million to 60 million people globally are affected by DFUs, a marked increase from 2015 estimates that ranged from 9 million to 26 million. Prevalence estimates vary widely and are influenced by differences in definitions of DFUs, the approach to surveillance, completeness of follow-up, and the definition of and approach to defining diabetes. A recent meta-analysis found a 6.3% global prevalence of DFUs among adults with diabetes, which equates to approximately 33 million people affected by DFU. While DFU has historically been reported at the highest rates in North America, modern cohort studies find rates upwards of 15% in populations with diabetes in Africa and South America.[11] The global prevalence of DFU is reported to be lower in adults with Type 1 compared with Type 2 diabetes, which may reflect younger age and cumulative duration, differences in study design and data collection, and/or lack of representative cohorts of people with Type 1 diabetes (T1D). A reminder of the importance of preventing DFUs in any part in the world is to remind ourselves that most diabetic amputations begin with a DFU.[12] Individuals with a closed DFU have high risk for recurrence, and should be considered as being in a state of remission.[13]

DIABETIC FOOT ULCERATION IN TYPES 1 AND 2 DIABETES

Generally, people with Type 2 diabetes are more likely to develop diabetic foot ulcers compared to those with T1D.[11] This higher incidence is primarily due to the fact that Type 2 diabetes is more prevalent and often associated with other risk factors such as obesity, peripheral vascular disease, and neuropathy, which increase the risk of developing foot ulcers.[14] Often, due to the associated neuropathy, the patient is unaware of the presence and extent of the ulcer even if there are signs of infection including purulence, fever, and signs of early sepsis. This is why patient education is so important regarding daily self-inspection of the foot, since the longer it takes to begin treatment, the greater risk there is for tissue loss, disability, osteomyelitis, sepsis, amputation, or death.[15]

In T1D, foot ulcers are less common but can still occur, especially in individuals with long-standing diabetes or poorly controlled blood sugar levels reflected by high A1C levels. Proper foot care and regular monitoring are essential in both types of diabetes for prevention and early detection of foot ulcers.

Many people consider Type I and Type 2 diabetes to be 2 different diseases but recent studies have suggested that they are both parts of a spectrum that may include autoimmune elements. Brooks-Worrell proposes that diabetes mellitus encompasses a spectrum of diseases with immune system involvement.[16] At one end of the spectrum are patients with classic childhood Type 1 disease encompassing autoimmune-mediated destructionof β cells. At the other end of the spectrum is Type 2 diabetes caused by a combination of defective insulin secretion by pancreatic β-cells and the inability of insulin-sensitive tissues to respond appropriately to insulin.[17]

PATHOPHYSIOLOGY OF DIABETIC FOOT ULCERS

Diabetic ulcers can be classified as neuropathic, ischemic, or combination neuro-ischemic. Diabetic foot ulcers comprise a full-thickness wound located in the weight-bearing or exposed area below the ankle. The Wagner System aids in categorizing the severity of the ulcer, ranking it on a scale of 1 to 5. Because of limitations of the Wagner System, a revised system was designed at the University of Texas, which includes vascularity and infection; making it an improved clinical tool (**Box 1**).[5,18]

Sensory neuropathy predisposes diabetic patients to induced upregulation of aldose reductase and sorbitol dehydrogenase, which in turn increases the production of fructose and sorbitol. These glucose products accumulate and induce osmotic stress, thereby reducing nerve cell myoinositol synthesis and nerve conduction. Increased advanced glycation end products (AGEs) present in diabetes also accelerate tissue damage.[18] In addition to sensory neuropathy, diabetes can induce autonomic dysfunction that results in impaired sweat production, leaving the foot susceptible to dryness, skin cracking, and fissuring. Furthermore, motor neuron dysfunction can give rise to muscle wasting and structural abnormalities of the foot. This causes focally elevated pressures at various zones of the plantar foot and increases the risk of ulceration.

Impaired wound healing is a key aspect of DFU progression. Molecular changes at the site of early DFU precede visualized tissue abnormalities. In the early phases of wound healing, neutrophils normally release granular molecules to kill foreign pathogens in a process known as neutrophil extracellular traps (NETosis). However, in a diabetic microenvironment, NETosis becomes dysregulated, causing a proinflammatory cascade and overproduction of cytokines and superoxide, which delays wound healing. Moreover, hyperglycemia induces formation of AGEs that cause structural and

---

Box 1
The University of Texas (UT) modified Wagner classification of DFU

The UT diabetic wound classification system

The grades of the UT system include:
- Grade 0: Pre- or post-ulcerative site (epithelialized wound)
- Grade 1: Superficial wound, not involving tendon, capsule, or bone
- Grade 2: Wound is penetrating to tendon or capsule
- Grade 3: Wound is penetrating bone or joint

There are 4 stages within each wound grade:
- Stage A: Clean wounds (no infection, no ischemia)
- Stage B: Nonischemic, infected wounds
- Stage C: Ischemic, noninfected wounds
- Stage D: Ischemic and infected wounds (both present)

From Boulton AJM, Whitehouse RW. The Diabetic Foot. [Updated 2023 Jul 28]. In: Feingold KR, Anawalt B, Blackman MR, et al., editors. Endotext [Internet]. South Dartmouth (MA): MDText.com, Inc.; 2000-. Figure 2. [The University of Texas Wound Classification System.]. Available from: https://www.ncbi.nlm.nih.gov/books/NBK409609/figure/diab-foot.F2/.

functional changes in key proteins. Ultimately, cytokine release is enhanced with a self-sustaining cascade that prolongs inflammation and favors apoptosis (cell death). Overall, hyperglycemia induces a proinflammatory environment largely due to the dysregulation of cytokine release, NETosis, and AGE production.[5]

Along with inflammation, alterations of the extracellular matrix (ECM) play a significant role in perpetuating the non-healing DFU. In normal wound healing, the production and degradation of ECM proteins such as collagen and fibrin are tightly regulated. Collagen comprises most of the soft tissue ECM, and abnormalities of collagen metabolism have significant consequences on wound healing. Specifically, collagen-degrading enzymes known as matrix metalloproteinases (MMPs) become hyperactive, resulting in a highly proteolytic environment with reduced collagen content. Overall, the ECM becomes disorganized and insufficient to support wound healing. Alongside elevated MMP activity, the accumulation of AGEs results in a reduction of fibroblast with growth factor (FGF) and transforming growth factor-beta. This has a similar effect of reducing collagen content via the induction of fibroblast apoptosis.

Lastly, impaired angiogenesis (new capillary formation) plays a key role in the disruption of diabetic wound healing.[19] Angiogenesis ordinarily occurs during the proliferative phase of wound healing and is responsible for both formation of granulation tissue and delivery of nutrition and oxygen to the wound. In the case of DFUs, there is a reduction of angiogenic growth factors such as vascular endothelial growth factor (VEGF) and FGF-2.[20] Vascular endothelial growth factor initiates angiogenesis and mediates endothelial cell proliferation while FGF-2 facilitates migration of new blood vessels through the ECM. When VEGF and FGF-2 expression is compromised, wound healing declines. Furthermore, endothelial progenitor cells (EPCs) have been implicated as expressors of proangiogenic factors and receptors including VEGF and FGF. A deficiency of function and number of EPCs has been demonstrated in patients with type 2 diabetes mellitus, which is attributed to AGE accumulation. Overall, the dysfunction of EPCs and circulating growth factors contributes significantly to development and progression of DFU by way of disrupting angiogenesis.

Central to the pathophysiology of DFUs are the neuropathy and angiopathy associated with diabetes, with contribution from comorbidities including renal disease, impairment of the immune system, and dysfunctional metabolic pathways due to insulin absence or dysfunction.[21] A consistent observation is the relationship between microvascular disease and peripheral neuropathy. Microvascular disease may contribute to diabetic neuropathy, including sensory, motor, and autonomic, and subcategories of those nerve types. There is much yet to discover about diabetic neuropathy and future research may open new pathways of diagnostic and therapeutic approaches for aging populations worldwide.

A PREVENTIVE, DIAGNOSTIC, AND THERAPEUTIC PLAN FOR HEALING

When acute wounds stray from the normal healing trajectory, they become chronic, which can lead to localized, then spreading infection, deepening wounds, sepsis, limb-threatening infections, amputation, and death. The role of the wound care practitioner is to create an environment of prevention through patient education, and when a wound does occur, apply a systematic process to assess the wound and develop a plan to heal that wound with minimal loss of tissue and function.

Before the advent of clinical practice guidelines, randomized controlled trial data, and updated diagnostic and treatment methodologies, wound care was based on trial and error with many products, which had no solid science to validate efficacy or cost-effectiveness. Today's world of wound care has improved, although new products continue to appear with claims of effectiveness based on weak evidence.[22] The authors still have a long way to go, with improved direction to construct clinical trials for products, devices, and surgical procedures that have the most promise.[23]

A "Plan for Healing" involves many different levels including evidence-based clinical practice guidelines, and involves knowledge, surgical skills, products, devices, and experience that will maximize healing outcomes.[24] The value of experience alone should never be underestimated, considering that a seasoned wound caregiver can draw on similar situations to find alternative pathways for healing. A team approach to healing DFU includes podiatric surgery, plastic surgery, vascular surgery, endovascular cardiology, general surgery, internal medicine, endocrinology, and anesthesiologists with knowledge of local and regional anesthesia.[25]

A Plan for Healing begins with a thorough history and physical, relevant laboratory values and diagnostics, assessing the patient's psychosocial situation and goals of care, and examination of the wound followed by application of evidenced-based clinical practice guidelines (preventive, diagnostic, and therapeutic), management of contributing co-morbidities, medical and surgical plans, and patient and family education.[26] A Plan for Healing is multifaceted, with many sources of information considered in deciding what a patient needs to heal, pathways to achieve that goal, and specific combination of procedures, products, devices, and specialty care that will provide the optimal outcome. A Plan for Healing also includes constant vigilance and enforcement of compliance, early identification of complications, and modified plans for healing based on evolving condition of the wound.

Total contact casting (TCC) is the treatment of choice for Wagner I and II diabetic foot ulcers, as it helps to promote healing by creating a more conducive environment for tissue repair.[27,28] The primary goal of TCC is to offload pressure from the ulcer site, which helps to reduce inflammation, minimize tissue damage, and promote the formation of healthy new tissue. Additionally, the cast provides stability to the foot and ankle, which can help to prevent further damage and promote proper healing. TCC involves encasing the foot and ankle in a specialized cast that evenly distributes pressure across the entire foot, thereby reducing pressure on the ulcerated area. By redistributing the weight-bearing forces away from the ulcer, TCC helps promote healing by creating a more conducive environment for tissue repair.

PATIENT ASSESSMENT

A history for a geriatric wound patient encompasses medical, surgical, and pharmacologic elements to optimize host factors to manage wound healing. The caregiver must understand those diseases, medications, and previous surgical procedures that can impact wound healing outcomes with vigilance for early detection of infection. Other considerations include cognitive, nutritional, and functional status. This requires systematic communication with the family, primary care physician, and other specialists caring for the patient's comorbidities to ensure optimal management of host factors necessary for healing.

The following questions should be considered when examining a geriatric patient and considering the diagnostic studies:

1. Is there an acute component to the wound?
2. Is there a chronic component to the wound?
3. Are there signs and symptoms of infection?
4. Are there signs and symptoms of ischemia?
5. Are there signs and symptoms of neuropathy?
6. What is the cognitive and psychosocial status of the patient?

7. Can this wound be healed, and is this wound considered palliative?

The value of a thorough wound–patient history and physical examination cannot be understated. After history and physical examination, there are considerations for diagnostics, then differential diagnosis with subspecialty second opinions when needed.[29] Further diagnostic studies can be added by consultants, culminating in a working diagnosis or diagnoses, particularly in the presence of comorbidities that can affect wound healing outcomes. Pain assessment in diabetics, particularly in the context of diabetic neuropathy or foot ulcers, requires a comprehensive approach due to its multifactorial nature.[30]

Physical examination should include palpation of pulses, capillary refill time, monofilament screen for sensation, and description and measurement of the wound including determining if the wound probes to bone. Diagnostics include laboratory tests such as complete blood count (CBC) and chemistries including serum albumin and HbA1C. Noninvasive vascular assessments include pulse volume recordings, transcutaneous oxygen tension, and others depending upon the capability of your local vascular laboratory. Ankle-brachial index measurement is unreliable in geriatric populations due to the high incidence of non-compressible arteries resulting in aberrant results. Diagnosis of osteomyelitis is best made through MRI, but bone biopsy offers more information by providing culture results to direct antibiotic therapy.[31]

Box 2 presents elements of a Plan for Healing. The plan has many elements; the absence of any one can reduce the healing outcome and functional rehabilitation.

PSYCHOSOCIAL AND QUALITY OF LIFE CONSIDERATIONS

Often, the effects on quality of life (QoL) are significant, both physically and mentally, among geriatric diabetic patients with some form of amputation, including partial

---

Box 2
Elements of a Plan for Healing

- Evaluation of arterial and venous disease with appropriate diagnostic studies
- Evaluation of wound and peri-wound: necrotic tissue, infection, and inflammatory tissue
- Evaluation of dysfunction and deformity
- Psychosocial and neurologic evaluation
- Evaluation of pain
- Evaluation of edema and lymphedema
- Evaluation of the wound bed microenvironment
- Laboratory assessment including CBC and HbA1C
- Strategies for optimizing tissue growth with advanced healing modalities
- Strategies for wound pressure relief by off-loading and wound immobilization
- Appropriate consultations including second opinions
- Treatment, follow-up, and healing maintenance
- Consideration of wishes of patient and family/POA
- Nutritional counseling and patient education
- Comprehensive post-discharge instructions with wound treatment and follow-up
- Plan for preventive foot care with continued patient education
- Determination of prognosis for healing

foot, or more proximal leg amputation.[32,33] In order to formulate a comprehensive treatment strategy, caregivers must consider the psychologic consequences of wounds and QoL. This will assist not only in determining feasibility of specific treatment decisions but also assist in prognostication and communication with the patient and family. Diabetic foot ulcers can result in mobility limitations with the need for environmental adaptations, with psychosocial consequences that include social isolation, financial hardship, and negative emotional states such as anxiety and depression. Any factor leading to nutritional deficit, including poverty, living alone, lack of access to food and safe drinking water, neuropsychologic problems, and medical issues such as malabsorbtion will impair healing and interrupt the Plan for Healing.

THE FUTURE

Given the increasing number of acute and chronic wounds in all countries worldwide, there is a need for enhanced medical and nursing school curricula, which includes the pathophysiology and clinical science of wound healing, including prevention, diagnosis, and treatment.[34] Considering that many patients contact their primary caregiver when they notice a new wound, there is a need to ensure proper diagnosis with improved referral patterns to wound specialists. Biomarkers are on the horizon for early identification of DFU and predictors of healing.[35,36]

Telemedicine has been used to monitor wound progress, reducing the expense of transportation for follow-up physician, and nursing care.[37] Telemedicine, combined with artificial intelligence (AI) can potentially provide preventive, diagnostic, and therapeutic interventions while reducing transportation for caregivers in remote locations. Artificial intelligence could assist caregivers to determine proper venues for medical and surgical care, plan diagnostics, and arrange patient transportation.[38]

There is a need to package educational information in pocket guides for wound clinicians on smart phones, including instructional videos, narrated presentations in multiple languages, live and archived conferences, and journal articles on all aspects of prevention, diagnosis, and treatment of wounds. Considering the rapid increase in diabetes worldwide, there is a need for global education on prevention, healing, and early detection of complications, with emphasis on the importance of the team approach.[4]

DIABETIC FOOT ULCER PREVENTION AND TREATMENT RESOURCES

The following are useful links to resources for prevention, treatment, and clinical practice guidelines for diabetic foot ulcers.

Diabetes support resources from the American Diabetic Association
https://professional.diabetes.org/diabetes-support-resources.

Clinical practice Guidelines from the International Working Group on the Diabetic Foot (IWGDF)
https://iwgdfguidelines.org/.

The management of diabetic foot: A clinical practice guideline by the Society for Vascular Surgery in collaboration with the American Podiatric Medical Association and the Society for Vascular Medicine
https://www.jvascsurg.org/article/S0741-5214(15)02025-X/fulltext.

CLINICS CARE POINTS

- The wound care practitioner must understand the diseases, medications, and prior and future surgical procedures that can impact wound healing outcomes.

- There should be systematic communication with the primary caregiver and specialists to ensure optimal management of host factors necessary for healing.
- Caregivers should be aware of medications that inhibit wound healing including corticosteroids, antineoplastics, and immunomodulators.
- Patients should be educated on prevention, including deleterious impact of lifestyle choices including obesity, smoking, drug, and alcohol abuse.
- Many wounds require multiple debridements to reduce necrotic tissue and biofilm and resolve infection.
- Debrided tissue needs time to revascularize through angiogenesis and edema should be minimized in preparation for primary closure or grafting to optimize healing.
- Patients with a history of soft-tissue infection or osteomyelitis should be assessed for ongoing residual infection, including Brodie's Abscess and chronic refractory osteomyelitis.
- The prevention of recurrence is an important aspect of management. While most patients with DFUs heal within 1 year, the recurrence rate remains high. Individuals with a closed DFU should be considered as being in a state of remission.
- When healing is not expected, a conservative and palliative care approach is appropriate.

DISCLOSURE

The authors have nothing to disclose.

REFERENCES

1. Greenfield G, Shmueli L, Harvey A, et al. Patient-initiated second medical consultations-patient characteristics and motivating factors, impact on care and satisfaction: a systematic review. BMJ Open 2021;11(9):e044033.
2. Miranda C, Da Ros R, Marfella R. Update on prevention of diabetic foot ulcer. Arch Med Sci Atheroscler Dis 2021;6:e123–31.
3. Lim JZ, Ng NS, Thomas C. Prevention and treatment of diabetic foot ulcers. J R Soc Med 2017;110(3):104–9.
4. Sen CK. Human wound and its burden: updated 2020 compendium of estimates. Adv Wound Care 2021;10(5):281–92.
5. Armstrong DG, Tan TW, Boulton AJM, et al. Diabetic foot ulcers: a review. JAMA 2023;330(1):62–75.
6. Armstrong DG, Boulton AJM, Bus SA. Diabetic foot ulcers and their recurrence. N Engl J Med 2017;376(24):2367–75.
7. Schmidt BM, Holmes CM. Updates on diabetic foot and Charcot osteopathic arthropathy. Curr Diab Rep 2018;18(10):74.
8. Raja JM, Maturana MA, Kayali S, et al. Diabetic foot ulcer: a comprehensive review of pathophysiology and management modalities. World J Clin Cases 2023;11(8):1684–93.
9. Akkus G, Sert M. Diabetic foot ulcers: a devastating complication of diabetes mellitus continues non-stop in spite of new medical treatment modalities. World J Diabetes 2022;13(12):1106–21.
10. Serena TE. A global perspective on wound care. Adv Wound Care 2014;3(8):548–52.
11. McDermott K, Fang M, Boulton AJM, et al. Etiology, epidemiology, and disparities in the burden of diabetic foot ulcers. Diabetes Care 2023;46(1):209–21.

12. Barnes JA, Eid MA, Creager MA, et al. Epidemiology and risk of amputation in patients with diabetes mellitus and peripheral artery disease. Arterioscler Thromb Vasc Biol 2020;40(8):1808–17.
13. Bouly M, Laborne FX, Tourte C, et al. Post-healing follow-up study of patients in remission for diabetic foot ulcers Pied-REM study. PLoS One 2022;17(5): e0268242. https://doi.org/10.1371/journal.pone.0268242.
14. Musa HG, Ahmed ME. Associated risk factors and management of chronic diabetic foot ulcers exceeding 6 months' duration. Diabet Foot Ankle 2012;3. https://doi.org/10.3402/dfa.v3i0.18980.
15. Rismayanti IDA, Nursalam N, Farida VN, et al. Early detection to prevent foot ulceration among type 2 diabetes mellitus patient: a multi-intervention review. J Public Health Res 2022;11(2):2752.
16. Brooks-Worrell BM, Tjaden AH, Edelstein SL, et al. Islet autoimmunity in adults with impaired glucose tolerance and recently diagnosed, treatment naïve type 2 diabetes in the restoring insulin SEcretion (RISE) study. Front Immunol 2021; 12:640251. https://doi.org/10.3389/fimmu.2021.640251.
17. Rajkumar V. and Levine S.N., Latent autoimmune diabetes, In: *StatPearls [Internet]*, 2024, StatPearls Publishing; Treasure Island (FL). Available at: https://www.ncbi.nlm.nih.gov/books/NBK557897/.
18. Yazdanpanah S, Rabiee M, Tahriri M, et al. Evaluation of glycated albumin (GA) and GA/HbA1c ratio for diagnosis of diabetes and glycemic control: a comprehensive review. Crit Rev Clin Lab Sci 2017;54(4):219–32.
19. Rai V, Moellmer R, Agrawal DK. Stem cells and angiogenesis: implications and limitations in enhancing chronic diabetic foot ulcer healing. Cells 2022;11(15): 2287.
20. Burgess JL, Wyant WA, Abdo Abujamra B, et al. Diabetic wound-healing science. Medicina (Kaunas) 2021;57(10):1072.
21. Hicks CW, Selvin E. Epidemiology of peripheral neuropathy and lower extremity disease in diabetes. Curr Diab Rep 2019;19(10):86.
22. Boulton AJM, Armstrong DG, Londahl M, et al. New evidence-based therapies for complex diabetic foot wounds. ADA Clinical Compendia 2022;2022(2):1–23.
23. Mavrogenis AF, Megaloikonomos PD, Antoniadou T, et al. Current concepts for the evaluation and management of diabetic foot ulcers. EFORT Open Rev 2018;3(9):513–25.
24. Senneville É, Albalawi Z, van Asten SA, et al. IWGDF/IDSA guidelines on the diagnosis and treatment of diabetes-related foot infections (IWGDF/IDSA 2023). Diabetes Metab Res Rev 2023;1:e3687. https://doi.org/10.1002/dmrr. 3687.
25. Musuuza J, Sutherland BL, Kurter S, et al. A systematic review of multidisciplinary teams to reduce major amputations for patients with diabetic foot ulcers. J Vasc Surg 2020;71(4):1433–46.e3.
26. Wang A, Lv G, Cheng X, et al. Guidelines on multidisciplinary approaches for the prevention and management of diabetic foot disease (2020 edition). Burns Trauma 2020;8:tkaa017.
27. McGuire JB. Pressure redistribution strategies for the diabetic or at-risk foot: part I. Adv Skin Wound Care 2006;19(4):213–21.
28. McGuire JB. Pressure redistribution strategies for the diabetic or at-risk foot: Part II. Adv Skin Wound Care 2006;19(5):270–7, quiz 277-9.
29. Hingorani A, LaMuraglia GM, Henke P, et al. The management of diabetic foot: a clinical practice guideline by the society for vascular surgery in collaboration with

the American podiatric medical association and the society for vascular medicine. J Vasc Surg 2016;63(2 Suppl):3S–21S.

30. Frescos N, Copnell B. Podiatrists' views of assessment and management of pain in diabetes-related foot ulcers: a focus group study. J Foot Ankle Res 2020; 13(1):29.

31. Lipsky BA, Berendt AR, Deery HG, et al, Infectious Diseases Society of America. Diagnosis and treatment of diabetic foot infections. Plast Reconstr Surg 2006; 117(7 Suppl):212S–38S.

32. Enweluzo GO, Asoegwu CN, Ohadugha AGU, et al. Quality of life and life after amputation among amputees in Lagos, Nigeria. J West Afr Coll Surg 2023; 13(3):71–6.

33. Calabrese L, Maffoni M, Torlaschi V, et al. What is hidden behind amputation? Quanti-qualitative systematic review on psychological adjustment and quality of life in lower limb amputees for non-traumatic reasons. Healthcare (Basel) 2023; 11(11):1661.

34. Yim E, Sinha V, Diaz SI, et al. Wound healing in US medical school curricula. Wound Repair Regen 2014;22(4):467–72.

35. Wang Y, Shao T, Wang J, et al. An update on potential biomarkers for diagnosing diabetic foot ulcer at early stage. Biomed Pharmacother 2021;133:110991. https://doi.org/10.1016/j.biopha.2020.110991.

36. Prasad Mahindrakar B, Goswami AG, Huda F, et al. Wound pH and surface temperature as a predictive biomarker of healing in diabetic foot ulcers. Int J Low Extrem Wounds 2023;22:15347346231156962.

37. Søndergaard SF, Vestergaard EG, Andersen AB, et al. How patients with diabetic foot ulcers experience telemedicine solutions: a scoping review. Int Wound J 2023;20(5):1796–810.

38. Chemello G, Salvatori B, Morettini M, et al. Artificial intelligence methodologies applied to technologies for screening, diagnosis and care of the diabetic foot: a narrative review. Biosensors 2022;12(11):985.

Other Wounds Encountered in Clinical Practice

Scott Matthew Bolhack, MD, MBA, CMD, CWSP, PCWC

KEYWORDS

- Pyoderma gangrenosum • Sickle cell disease ulcers • Vasculitic wounds
- Martorell hypertensive ischemic leg ulcers • Wounds associated with malignancy

KEY POINTS

- This article delves into atypical wounds encountered by wound care clinicians, encompassing conditions such as pyoderma gangrenosum, sickle cell disease–related wounds, Martorell hypertensive ischemic leg ulcers, vasculitis-associated wounds, and those linked to malignancy.
- Prevalence data for these wounds are limited, and their occurrence often depends on the clinical setting and referral patterns.
- The diagnostic process for atypical wounds involves the use of algorithms, clinical experience, and testing, with skin biopsies being a crucial tool.
- Collaboration with specialists is common due to the complex nature of these wounds, with experienced clinicians identifying underlying disorders and initiating referrals.

OVERVIEW

In addition to usual wounds that the wound care clinician encounters (venous, arterial, neuropathic, pressure, surgical, lymphatic), there are a multitude of less common wounds. Atypical wounds are unusual presentations of any wound type. Most wounds encountered in clinical practice cannot be considered "rare," since there are few references that measure prevalence of these wounds. The general experience by wound clinicians for less commonly seen wounds is also a function of where the clinician practices or what types of referrals are made to the clinician in their specific setting.

This article will review wounds due to pyoderma gangrenosum (PG), sickle cell disease (SCD), Martorell hypertensive ischemic leg ulcers, wounds associated with vasculitis, and wounds due to malignancy. There are numerous other wounds that a dedicated wound specialist will see over their career, so this article will not exhaust all uncommon wounds that one will see.

There are many algorithms that the wound clinician utilizes to make a diagnosis and create a treatment plan. Along with clinical experience, testing is a key component to

TLC HealthCare Wound Consultants, 1775 East Skyline Drive, #101, Tucson, AZ 85718, USA
E-mail address: sbolhack@gmail.com

Clin Geriatr Med 40 (2024) 449–458
https://doi.org/10.1016/j.cger.2024.03.012
0749-0690/24/© 2024 Elsevier Inc. All rights reserved.

geriatric.theclinics.com

assist the clinician in making the correct diagnosis. Uncommon and atypical wounds often involve a skin biopsy, an important diagnostic tool for the wound care clinician. Access to a dermatopathologist is important for making an accurate diagnosis. Often, the biopsy helps the clinician rule out other considerations without an exact finding for the specific diagnosis, and repeating a biopsy or multiple biopsies may be necessary.

The timing of a biopsy can also be important. A biopsy of a wound is warranted when there is no healing despite treating the underlying etiology. While some text-books suggest that a wound be biopsied after a certain length of time, wound clini-cians often see patients after many weeks to months (years) of nonhealing but without interventions addressing the underlying etiology. Experience and judgment are vital, and depending on setting, a biopsy may not be possible and referral to a specialist with biopsy capabilities is necessary. Many uncommon wounds require specific laboratory testing to aid in the diagnosis, especially with wounds associated with the vasculitis.

Due to the nature of these wounds, collaboration with other specialists will be the norm, not the exception. An experienced wound clinician may be the first to suggest an underlying disorder and will refer the patient to the specialist. However, more commonly, the patient is sent to the wound clinician from the specialist with an estab-lished diagnosis with a complication of a wound as part of the disease process.

PYODERMA GANGRENOSUM

PG is a rare, inflammatory, and rapidly progressive skin disorder that is often difficult to diagnose and treat (**Fig. 1**). The wound is characterized by features of painful, necrotic skin ulcers that are unresponsive to standard wound care measures. PG is associated with systemic conditions such as inflammatory bowel disease, rheumatoid arthritis, and hematologic malignancies; but often an underlying disorder cannot be determined.

The diagnosis of PG can be challenging, as it can present with similar clinical fea-tures to other necrotic skin disorders. The diagnosis is based on clinical criteria, including the characteristic ulcer morphology, the rapid progression of the ulcer, and the exclusion of other causes of ulceration, such as infection or malignancy.[1–3] Pathergy is the characteristic condition where an exaggerated and intensely painful skin lesion arises secondarily to minor trauma such as scratches, bumps, and

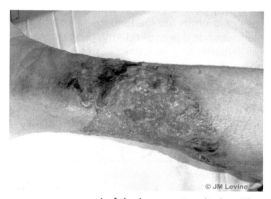

Fig. 1. Pyoderma gangrenosum wound of the lower extremity in a 72-year-old woman. This wound exhibited the phenomenon of "pathergy" whereby a small trauma elicited a large painful wound. (*Courtesy of* Jeffrey M. Levine, MD, AGSF, CMD.)

excisional debridement. Histologic examination of skin biopsy samples can aid in the diagnosis, as PG is characterized by a dense inflammatory infiltrate composed of neutrophils and mononuclear cells. Providing photographs and communicating with the pathologist can assist in making the diagnosis.

The treatment of PG involves a multidisciplinary approach, including local wound care, anti-inflammatory therapies, and treatment of the underlying systemic condition. Sharp excisional debridement of the wound can aggravate the inflammatory process, so a conservative approach is desired. Topical agents, such as corticosteroids and calcineurin inhibitors, may be useful in mild cases, while systemic immunosuppressive agents, such as glucocorticoids, cyclosporine, and azathioprine, are used in more severe cases.[4] Biologic agents, such as infliximab, adalimumab, and rituximab, have also shown promise in the treatment of PG.[5]

The management of PG is challenging and requires close monitoring of the wound and the patient's underlying systemic condition. The use of a multidisciplinary team, including a dermatologist, rheumatologist, and wound care specialist, will assist in optimal management.

The prognosis of PG is variable and depends on the severity of the ulcer, underlying systemic condition, and the response to treatment. In some cases, PG may be self-limiting, and the ulcer may heal spontaneously. In more severe cases, PG can result in significant morbidity, including limb amputation and even death.[6] Early diagnosis and aggressive management are crucial for improving outcomes in patients with PG.

In summary, PG is a rare and challenging disorder that requires a multidisciplinary approach for optimal management. Diagnosis is based on clinical criteria, and treatment involves wound care, anti-inflammatory therapies, and treatment of the underlying systemic condition. Prognosis is variable and depends on the severity of the ulcer and the response to treatment. Physicians should be aware of PG and consider it in the differential diagnosis of necrotic skin ulcers in patients with underlying systemic conditions.

SICKLE CELL DISEASE ULCERATIONS

SCD, the most prevalent global hemoglobinopathy, particularly affects individuals of sub-Saharan African, Mediterranean, Indian, and Middle Eastern ancestry. SCD includes any of the syndromes associated with the sickle mutation co-inherited with a mutation at the other betaglobin allele. Patients with just the sickle cell trait are not at risk for these types of ulcerations.

The complications of SCD are related to hemolytic anemia and vaso-occlusion which leads to pain, tissue ischemia, and infarction. The risk of infection is increased due to functional hyposplenism from splenic infarction. Leg ulcers are a common complication of SCD. The pathophysiology of the ulcer formation has not been completely elucidated. The ulcers are seen more in males, after the age of 10. Typical sites are the medial and lateral malleoli. Leg ulcers, a persistent issue in SCD, pose significant challenges, often healing slowly and recurring over extended periods, and detrimentally affecting quality of life.

With the appearance of a leg ulcer, a lower extremity venous Doppler to evaluate for deep vein thrombosis (DVT) is recommended as 44% of leg ulcers in patients with SCD are associated with DVT.[7] Since pulmonary hypertension is associated with the development of lower extremity ulcers, referral to a pulmonologist is recommended.

Management of the wound will involve multiple disciplines. No specific wound treatments for ulcers associated with SCD have been shown to be beneficial.[8] Systemic treatments with hydroxyurea and transfusions will likely be required.[9] Local wound care with compression is recommended when edema is associated with the development of these wounds. The patient with SCD may have multiple factors that make healing of these leg ulcers challenging including malnutrition, nutritional deficiencies, pulmonary hypertension, pain, and depression.

VASCULITIC WOUNDS

A patient with underlying vasculitis can present with a spectrum of dermatologic manifestations, including wounds. Most of the skin presentations of vasculitis (nodules, purpura, discoloration of the gums, urticarial papules, petechiae, livedo racemosa) will not be the reason that the patient is referred to the wound specialist; however, once there are hemorrhagic bullae or open wounds, the practitioner should be aware of the coexistence of these other skin manifestations that can lead to the diagnosis of vasculitis. Almost all patients that present with vasculitis to the wound center with an ulcer will have some systemic manifestation of the specific underlying vasculitis.

The combination of laboratory testing and skin biopsies, along with a high index of suspicion for underlying vasculitis, is necessary as these wounds can mimic other commonly seen wounds. The involvement of a dermatologist, rheumatologist, allergist, immunologist, and dermatopathologist is often necessary to make the correct diagnosis. The finding on the biopsy of inflammation and damage to the blood vessel walls is confirmatory.[10] With ulcers that are suspect for vasculitis, a punch biopsy should be taken along the edge of the ulcer. The timing and location of the biopsy taken are important to making the correct diagnosis. Typically, leukocytoclastic vasculitis is observed with infiltration of arterioles and postcapillary venules by neutrophils undergoing degranulation and fragmentation. There may also be fibrinoid necrosis of inflamed vessel in medium and small arteries of the reticular dermis and fat. Direct immunofluorescence can be helpful to confirm immunoglobulin and complement deposits.

Due to the numerous types of vasculitis, the overlapping associated symptoms, and variability of the disease presentation from patient to patient, generalities related to the clinical presentation of vasculitis ulcerations cannot be oversimplified. Most of the cutaneous vasculitis syndromes that can result in ulcerations are of the medium and small vessels. Shallow ulcerations are mostly associated with small-vessel vasculitis, which has a predilection for the lower extremities (cutaneous small-vessel vasculitis, granulomatosis with polyangiitis—also known as Wegener's granulomatosis), eosinophilic granulomatosis with polyangiitis (Churg-Strauss syndrome), microscopic polyangiitis, cryoglobulinemic vasculitis, and rheumatoid vasculitis. The medium-vessel vasculitis syndromes associated with ulcerations include polyarteritis nodosa, cutaneous polyarteritis nodosa, and nodular vasculitis. The urticarial forms of small-vessel vasculitis do not readily result in ulcerations of the skin (immunoglobulin A vasculitis/Henoch-Schönlein purpura, urticarial vasculitis, or cutaneous small-vessel vasculitis). Large-vessel vasculitis such as giant-cell arteritis, Takayasu arteritis, and relapsing polychondritis does not affect blood vessels in the skin, and are rarely a concern to the wound care clinician.[11]

Treatment for wounds associated with vasculitis requires an accurate diagnosis so the underlying vasculitis disorder is treated. Management requires collaboration with specialists. Wound care is largely supportive and the clinician should expect the wound to improve as the specific form of vasculitis is treated effectively.

Fig. 2 shows a left medial ankle wound in a 59 year-old woman with biopsy diagnosed as cutaneous small-vessel vasculitis. She initially presented with 9 wounds

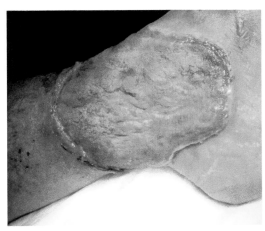

Fig. 2. Left medical ankle wound in a 59-year-old woman with biopsy diagnosed as cutaneous small-vessel vasculitis. (*Courtesy of* Scott Matthew Bolhack, MD, MBA, CMD, CWSP, PCWC, FACP.)

on the lower extremities. With systemic control and weekly wound care, it took over 2 years to completely heal all of her wounds.

MARTORELL HYPERTENSIVE ISCHEMIC LEG ULCER

A Martorell hypertensive ischemic ulcer (MHIU) is a complication of hypertension and medial calcification that can lead to limb-threatening ischemia and necrosis. The condition was first described in 1945 by Antoni Martorell, a Spanish pathologist who observed the presence of deep, painful ulcers in the legs of hypertensive patients.[12] The pathogenesis of Martorell ulcers is not fully understood. The MHIU was originally thought to be related to hypertension-induced vascular changes, including medial hypertrophy, intimal hyperplasia, and endothelial dysfunction. More recent studies show a relation to medial calcification of the small arterioles in the subcutaneous tissue.[13,14] This, in turn, results in tissue ischemia and necrosis, which manifests as the characteristic ulcer.

The diagnosis of MHIU is primarily clinical. These painful wounds appear mostly in middle-aged women on the lateral-dorsal lower extremities, and often present bilaterally. Due to the necrosis and pain, these wounds can be confused with PG, so differentiation is important as they require different treatments. A skin biopsy can aid in the diagnosis. Histologically, the ulcer is characterized by thrombosis of small arterioles and venules, with a surrounding inflammatory infiltrate. A Doppler ultrasound can help identify the presence of arteriovenous shunts and assess blood flow. 60% of patients were diabetic in one series.[14,15] An example of an MHIU in a 62-year-old woman appears in **Fig. 3**.

The treatment of an MHIU is challenging and requires a multidisciplinary approach, including blood pressure control, wound care, and surgical interventions. Blood pressure control is crucial and may involve aggressive antihypertensive therapy including intravenous vasodilators and continuous blood pressure monitoring. Wound care involves debridement, dressings, and offloading to reduce pressure on the ulcer. In severe cases, surgical intervention, such as arterial ligation or skin grafting, may be necessary.[14,16]

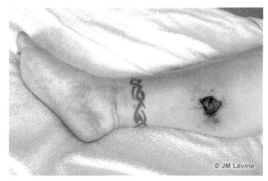

Fig. 3. Martorell's hypertensive ischemic ulcer in a 62-year-old woman. (*Courtesy of* Jeffrey M. Levine, MD, AGSF, CMD.)

The prognosis of an MHIU is poor, with a high risk of limb amputation and mortality. Early diagnosis and aggressive management may improve outcomes, but the rarity of this disorder and the lack of standard treatment guidelines make management challenging.

MALIGNANT ULCERS

The clinician will encounter patients with many forms of cancer including primary skin cancers where the presentation is atypical. Biopsies are the standard of care for making a diagnosis. Specific sources include primary skin tumors or metastatic lesions from breast, lung, head and neck, and genital malignancies. Malignant wounds can present as nodules, induration, fungating masses, malignant ulcers, zosteriform, and mixed appearance. **Fig. 4** shows the skin of an 87-year-old male who presented with an ulcerated melanoma of the foot. **Fig. 5** shows a malignant breast lesion on a 74-year-old female with cutaneous metastases and yellow malodorous drainage.

Basal cell, squamous cell, and melanoma cancers are sometimes missed by clinicians, and it is not until the patient is seen by the wound specialist in a later ulcerative phase of the cancer that a diagnosis is made. A careful history and a high index of

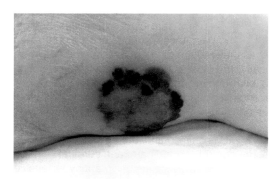

Fig. 4. An 87-year-old male presented with an ulcerated melanoma of the foot. (*Courtesy of* Scott Matthew Bolhack, MD, MBA, CMD, CWSP, PCWC, FACP.)

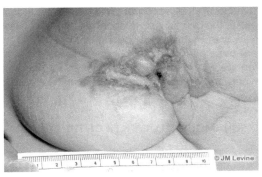

Fig. 5. Malignant breast lesion in a 74-year-old female. (*Courtesy of* Jeffrey M. Levine, MD, AGSF, CMD.)

suspicion lead to a biopsy of the wound to make the diagnosis. A keratoacanthoma (KA) is a form of squamous cell carcinoma that can present as a nonhealing wound. A characteristic of the KA is rapid lesion growth followed by quiescence and even by spontaneous resolution. The treatment of a KA is wide excisional biopsy with a 4 mm margin.

The wound clinician will encounter patients with fungating, malignant wounds. Rarely, these presentations are the initial opportunity to make a diagnosis; rather, these patients have already been diagnosed with cancer, and the wound care expert is asked to create a plan for management of the affected wound. Effective wound care for non-dermatologic malignancies requires a collaborative, interdisciplinary approach involving oncologists, plastic surgeons, wound care specialists, and nurses. By emphasizing patient education, support, and incorporating palliative care considerations, such a holistic approach addresses pain management and enhances overall quality of life. Understanding the expectations of the patient is the primary focus.

Discussions with the patient on the goals of wound care is vital (pain control, odor, debris and drainage control, ability to change dressings, cost of dressings, cure, and so forth). The clinician can simply ask the open-ended question to the patient: "What is bothering you most about your wound?" While these wounds are often the visible sign that the patient has a late-stage cancer, it should not prevent choices for treatments that would benefit the well-being of the patient. The use of limited surgery, radiation, or chemotherapy sometimes can be helpful in controlling the disease burden of an ulcerated cancerous wound. To the contrary, suggesting aggressive treatment options in patients with limited life expectancy is not prudent. Effective wound care requires a collaborative, interdisciplinary approach involving oncologists, plastic surgeons, wound care specialists, and nurses. By emphasizing patient education, support, and incorporating palliative care considerations, such a holistic approach addresses pain management and enhances overall quality of life.

Wounds related to cancer that present after radiation are challenging. Due to subclinical radiation dermatitis, the irradiated beds render the healing process difficult at a stage when cancer is often advanced. As with fungating cancerous wounds, discussions with the patient are necessary to establish the best goals for the patient.

A common presentation is a female with ulcerations in the field of radiation for breast cancer. The skin is the visible extension of the patient and their disease. It is one thing to know that you have a malignant process internally, but when this extends to the skin, this is a reminder of a disease process that has been difficult to eradicate let alone control. Covering up the wounds may hide the wounds from view, but the dressings themselves are the pervasive reminder that something is wrong. The patient may eventually pass away from the cancer but rarely from the wound itself. The intensity of the wound care required (dressing changes and wound care visits) often conflicts with the time required for the other visits required for chemotherapy, oncology, and primary care. Hyperbaric oxygen treatments can also be considered for radiation skin damage.[17]

CASE OF ADVANCED SQUAMOUS CELL CANCER OF THE CALVARIA AFTER RADIATION

A 73-year-old man was diagnosed with squamous cell cancer of the scalp. He was treated with surgery, then subsequent radiation. His initial presentation 5 years after initial treatments is seen in **Fig. 4**. He had exposed necrotic calvaria bone with a large pocket of exudate posteriorly under a skin flap.

The pocket of exudate was drained and cultured, and the patient was placed on antibiotics. The author removed as much of the necrotic tissue as safe in the wound center setting. Prior to the initial visit, the patient had been seen by his primary care physician, dermatologist, and oncologist. The radiation oncologist had not interacted with the patient for at least 2 years. After the first visit, we used alginate under the posterior skin flap; we crushed metronidazole and sprinkled it in the wound to control the odor. A call was made to the primary care physician to communicate findings and plan of care.

The patient was seen over the next 11 months with control of drainage and odor, which was his primary focus. By the end of the first month, when he was feeling better, he was thinking about seeking medical opinions for further treatments. When edges of the wound were biopsied, they revealed squamous cell cancer. In consultation with the oncologist and a surgeon that specializes in the reconstruction of head and neck cancers, it was agreed that he be treated palliatively. He lived his last 3 months under the care of hospice where the wound care was performed with a simplified dressing regimen.

CLINICS CARE POINTS

PG:
- Clinical criteria: Diagnose based on characteristic ulcer morphology, rapid progression, and exclusion of other causes.
- Collaboration is the key: Involve dermatologists, rheumatologists, and wound care specialists for accurate diagnosis and optimal management.
- Multidisciplinary treatment: Employ a range of therapies, including wound care and systemic agents, tailored to the severity of the ulcer and underlying conditions.

SCD ulcerations:
- Thrombosis assessment: Conduct a lower extremity venous Doppler to evaluate for deep vein thrombosis in patients with leg ulcers.
- Multidisciplinary management: Collaborate with pulmonologists and hematologists for comprehensive care addressing systemic and local factors.
- Expectation management: Acknowledge challenges in healing, recurrence, and quality of life in patients with persistent leg ulcers.

Vasculitic wounds:
- High index of suspicion: Recognize that vasculitis-associated ulcers may coexist with various skin manifestations, necessitating a thorough evaluation.

- Biopsy guidance: Utilize punch biopsies along the edge of ulcers for accurate diagnosis, considering timing and location.
- Specialist involvement: Collaborate with dermatologists, rheumatologists, allergists, immunologists, and dermatopathologists for a comprehensive diagnostic approach.

Martorell hypertensive ischemic leg ulcer:
- Clinical diagnosis: Diagnose based on clinical presentation, noting bilateral, painful ulcers in hypertensive patients.
- Vascular assessment: Use Doppler ultrasound to identify arteriovenous shunts and assess blood flow, aiding in confirmation.
- Multidisciplinary team: Involve blood pressure control, wound care, and surgical interventions in collaboration with various specialists.

Malignant ulcers:
- Biopsy vigilance: Conduct biopsies for suspicious wounds, especially when encountering atypical presentations of skin cancers.
- Interdisciplinary collaboration: Collaborate with oncologists, surgeons, and wound care specialists for optimal cancer management and wound care.
- Patient-centered care: Engage in discussions with patients to understand goals, addressing pain, odor control, and overall quality of life.

Radiation-related wounds
- Patient discussions: Engage in open conversations with patients regarding realistic goals for wound care postradiation.
- Holistic approach: Emphasize interdisciplinary collaboration, incorporating oncologists, plastic surgeons, and wound care specialists.
- Palliative considerations: Recognize the challenges of wound care in advanced cancer stages, aligning treatments with patient well-being.

DISCLOSURE

The authors have nothing to disclose.

REFERENCES

1. Su WP, Davis MD, Weenig RH, et al. Pyoderma gangrenosum: clinicopathologic correlation and proposed diagnostic criteria. Int J Dermatol 2004;43(11): 790–800.
2. Alavi A, French LE, Davis MD, et al. Pyoderma gangrenosum: an update on pathophysiology, diagnosis and treatment. Am J Clin Dermatol 2017;18(3):355–72.
3. Maverakis E, Ma C, Shinkai K, et al. Diagnostic criteria of ulcerative pyoderma gangrenosum: a Delphi consensus of international experts. JAMA Dermatol 2018;154(4):461–6.
4. Reichrath J, Bens G, Bonowitz A, et al. Treatment recommendations for pyoderma gangrenosum: an evidence-based review of the literature based on more than 350 patients. J Am Acad Dermatol 2005;53(2):273–83.
5. Brooklyn TN, Dunnill MG, Shetty A, et al. Infliximab for the treatment of pyoderma gangrenosum: a randomised, double-blind, placebo-controlled trial. Gut 2006; 55(4):505–9.
6. Binus AM, Qureshi AA, Li VW, et al. Pyoderma gangrenosum: a retrospective review of patient characteristics, comorbidities and therapy in 103 patients. Br J Dermatol 2011;165(6):1244–50.
7. Minniti CP, Delaney KM, Gorbach AM, et al. Vasculopathy, inflammation, and blood flow in leg ulcers of patients with sickle cell anemia. Am J Hematol 2014; 89(1):1–6.

8. Wun T, Hassell K. Best practices for transfusion for patients with sickle cell disease. Wun T, Hassell K. Hematol Rep 2009;1:e22.

9. Martí-Carvajal AJ, Knight-Madden JM, Martinez-Zapata MJ. Interventions for treating leg ulcers in people with sickle cell disease. Cochrane Database Syst Rev 2021 Jan 9;1(1):CD008394.

10. Carlson JA. The histological assessment of cutaneous vasculitis. Carlson JA Histopathology 2010;56(1):3.

11. Xu LY, Esparza EM, Anadkat MJ, et al. Cutaneous manifestations of vasculitis. Semin Arthritis Rheum 2009;38:348.

12. Martorell A. Multiple and recurrent spontaneous cutaneous hemorrhages of arteriovenous origin. Am J Pathol 1945;21:531–51.

13. Hafner J, Nobbe S, Partsch H, et al. Martorell hypertensive ischemic leg ulcer: a model of ischemic subcutaneous arteriolosclerosis. Arch Dermatol 2010;146(9): 961–8.

14. Shelling ML, Federman DG, Kirsner RS. Clinical approach to atypical wounds with a new model for understanding hypertensive ulcers. Arch Dermatol 2010 Sep;146(9):1026–9.

15. Vano-Galvan S, Hermosa-Gelbard Á, Fernández-Martínez R, et al. Martorell hypertensive ischemic leg ulcer: a review. Am J Clin Dermatol 2018;19(1):65–71.

16. Lima Pinto AP, Silva NA Jr, Osorio CT, et al. Martorell's ulcer: diagnostic and therapeutic challenge. Case Rep Dermatol 2015 Aug 5;7(2):199–206.

17. Cooper JS, Hanley ME, Hendriksen S, et al. Hyperbaric treatment of delayed radiation injury. In: StatPearls Internet. Treasure Island (FL): StatPearls Publishing; 2023. Available at: https://www.ncbi.nlm.nih.gov/books/NBK470447/.

Surgical Aspects of Wound Care in Older Adults

Lisa J. Gould, MD, PhD[a,b,*]

KEYWORDS

- Chronic wounds • Traumatic wounds • Skin grafts • Flap reconstruction
- Debridement • Prehabilitation • Older adult • Frailty

KEY POINTS

- Comorbid illness in older adults increases the complexity of surgical procedures.
- A team approach is critical to successful surgical treatment of wounds in older adults.
- Innovative approaches and surgical techniques can promote healing of complex wounds in older adults.
- Surgical closure of wounds can prevent hospital readmissions.

BACKGROUND: THE BURDEN OF WOUNDS IN OLDER ADULTS

Surgical treatment of wounds in older adults needs to consider the cause, severity, and likelihood of healing. In addition to chronic wounds, such as venous leg ulcers, diabetic foot ulcers, arterial insufficiency, and pressure injuries, older adults disproportionately experience skin tears, avulsion injuries from minor trauma, malignancy, and wound complications after surgical procedures.[1,2] In terms of expenditures, adults aged older than 65 years represent approximately 45% of the top 10% of health-care users and account for more than 40% of the surgical volume in the United States.[3] However, aside from expense to the health-care system, it is important to consider the full impact on the patient and caregivers, including direct costs from wound care supplies, hospital and nursing costs, indirect costs from lost wages that affect the patient and the unpaid caregivers, and intangible costs from pain, anxiety, loss of independence, reduced mobility, and exacerbation of concurrent illnesses.[4]

Surgical procedures in older adults are not to be taken lightly. Advances in anesthesia and postoperative care have enabled surgeons to successfully operate on patients aged older than 80 years.[5] Although many older people remain active in their later years, approximately 80% have at least one chronic condition and 75% have 2

[a] Department of Surgery, South Shore Health, Weymouth, MA, USA; [b] The Warren Alpert Medical School of Brown University, Providence, RI, USA
* Corresponding author. 90 Libbey Parkway, East Weymouth, MA 02189.
E-mail address: Lgould44@hotmail.com

Clin Geriatr Med 40 (2024) 459–470
https://doi.org/10.1016/j.cger.2023.12.012
0749-0690/24/© 2023 Elsevier Inc. All rights reserved.
geriatric.theclinics.com

or more.[6] This greatly influences the ability of older adults to cope with and heal a wound, whether it is acute or chronic. The most common wound type among patients aged older than 65 years is a surgical dehiscence, occurring in up to 30% of patients, complicated by mortality rates as high as 50%.[7,8] Any decision to operate must extend beyond the technical exercise, with an emphasis on evaluating the likelihood of successful recovery, especially the return to preoperative function. A holistic approach to risk stratification is even more important in older adults because this population is extremely heterogeneous. Illustrative of the complexity of patients with wounds, several studies of outpatient wound centers confirm that these patients have multiple comorbidities that impact wound healing, including malnutrition, diabetes, end-stage renal disease, hypertension, and venous insufficiency.[9-11] A recent study from a hospital-based outpatient wound center, in which approximately 50% of the patients were aged older than 65 years, determined that on average this real-world sample of patients had 8 comorbidities or conditions that would affect wound healing.[12] In addition to influencing the patient's quality of life, multimorbidity increases the likelihood of frailty by about 2-fold. As an indicator of the patient's mental and physiologic reserve, frailty in patients with wounds has been shown to correlate with increased hospital admissions, wound complications, and poor wound healing.[9] Studies of outpatient wound centers confirm that although there are many tools that have been used to measure frailty, most are too cumbersome to incorporate into the typical surgical preoperative assessment. Recent literature suggests that a 5-item frailty assessment (mFI-5) is a valuable screening tool and is prognostic of surgical outcomes.[13,14] Thus, in addition to chronologic age, an objective frailty index such as the mFI-5 not only provides insight into the patient's ability to heal and tolerate surgical procedures but can be a valuable tool for shared decision-making.

Wound treatment is complex in older adults because of the combination of age-impaired healing and the constellation of comorbid illnesses. Many factors enter into the decision-making process about whether a surgical approach will improve the outcome and promote more rapid healing. Wound clinicians need to consider that although a nonsurgical approach may lead to delayed healing, which increases the risk of infection, surgical treatment may not be necessary or provide overall benefit and may increase the risk of additional complications, especially in frail older adults.

DISCUSSION
Preoperative Assessment

The 4 Ms framework is an initiative of the Institute for Healthcare Improvement and the John A Hartford Foundation. Utilization of the 4 Ms to promote an Age Friendly Health System approach is critical when treating older adults, particularly when considering surgery. Overlapping but predating the 4 Ms is the Geriatric Surgery Verification (GSV) Program, which was created by a collaboration of the John A Hartford Foundation, the American College of Surgeons and multiple stakeholders. In addition to emphasizing goals and decision-making, cognition and preventing delirium, maintaining function and mobility, the GSV includes optimizing nutrition and hydration.[15] Because patients with wounds are medically complex, it is reasonable to coalesce these 2 initiatives when surgically treating wounds in older adults. All conversations regarding a surgical approach should start with asking, "What matters *most*?" to better understand the goals of the patient and set the stage for shared decision-making. This conversation will also discuss the anticipated impact of the operation, with a focus on symptoms, function, independence, and quality of life. Because most wound surgeries are relatively noninvasive (ie, not entering a body cavity), rather than discussing survival from the surgery, the conversation can focus on whether the surgery will ultimately impact long-term survival, reduce the need for future admissions, and decrease the likelihood of infections. In fact, the return to premorbid function and retention of functional independence is often what matters most to the older adult. Nonetheless, any surgery that requires a general anesthetic carries an increased risk in patients with multimorbidity, frailty, and/or dementia, all of which are common in older adults with wounds.

Medication is the second M of the 4 Ms. In addition to avoiding medications that are traditionally known to harm older adults, such as benzodiazepines, opioids, and anticholinergic medications, when considering an extensive wound debridement, it is critical to know whether the patient is anticoagulated and whether and when that anticoagulation can be held.[16] This entails a collaborative approach with the patient's primary care physician and/or cardiologist and may require some coordination to ensure appropriate timing of any intervention. Antibiotics are another class of medication that warrants review in the older adult. In addition to drug interactions, older adults are more susceptible to side effects related to age and changes in metabolism, development of multidrug-resistant infections, and *Clostridium difficile*. Antibiotic stewardship for wounds should follow the guidance of the International Wound Infection Institute.[17] By following these guidelines and using appropriately obtained wound or bone cultures, antibiotic use and the common adverse reactions that are prevalent in older adults will be reduced.

Mentation: Up to 37% of patients aged older than 60 years undergoing noncardiac elective surgery have baseline cognitive deficits that place them at higher risk of worsened postoperative cognitive dysfunction.[18] Deficits may range from mild cognitive impairment to dementia. Validated screening tests may be a valuable adjunct and signal the need to involve family members or other caregivers in conversations about surgical treatment and recovery. Assessment of the capacity for medical decision-making is nonnegotiable when evaluating geriatric patients. Many patients admitted with wounds that require surgery present with altered mental status, either from sepsis related to the wound or an alternative source. It may be difficult to evaluate the patient's baseline until there has been adequate source control.

Postoperative cognitive changes are one of the most common complications in older adults after general anesthetic but are often overlooked in preoperative discussions, especially when the deficit is subtle. Risk factors for postoperative cognitive dysfunction include preexisting cognitive decline, history of cerebrovascular accident, depression, age greater than 70 years, alcohol use, poor baseline functional status, and abnormal electrolytes; however, preoperative cognitive impairment is the risk factor most closely associated with developing postoperative delirium, which can lead to prolonged hospitalization, functional decline, long-term cognitive decline, and development of dementia.[19] Postoperative measures that can aid recovery and minimize delirium include using opioid-sparing multimodal analgesia and limiting anticholinergic medications, implementing early family or caregiver support, maintaining normal sleep–wake cycles, early mobilization if possible and returning sensory aids such as glasses and hearing aids as early as possible.[20]

Addressing the fourth M, mobility is one of the most difficult aspects of wound surgery. Impaired mobility is often one of the reasons that older adults have wounds that require surgery and many patients will require altered positioning or immobilization after surgery to heal the wound. A major consideration for flaps or grafts on the trunk, including pressure ulcer reconstruction, is the need for an extended period of bedrest to immobilize the surgical site. The detrimental effect of bedrest in older adults is well documented. In fact, physical inactivity is the fourth leading risk factor for global mortality.[21] If the procedure is truly elective, a period of prehabilitation in which the functional capability is improved to prepare the older adult for surgery is beneficial. This process, which includes an emphasis on nutritional supplementation, smoking cessation, physical and cognitive exercise, and stress reduction, may help the patient withstand the decline that accompanies postoperative inactivity.[22] However, if it is not possible to incorporate a period of prehabilitation, it has been shown that older adults can benefit from exercise during an acute hospitalization.[23] Even exercise in bed can improve overall conditioning and should be considered for patients undergoing flap reconstruction.[24]

Surgical procedures in older adults carry risks beyond cognitive changes. Advanced age combined with baseline comorbidities, especially a history of recent respiratory failure, can put patients at increased risk for what might be considered a "minor" surgery. A Medicare database review reported a 30-day mortality rate of 0.66% for outpatient surgery with increased risk for patients aged older than 85 years.[25,26] Thus, an interprofessional team that includes the anesthesiologist, surgeons, and others involved in the patient's care to minimize risk and maximize recovery is essential. Ideally, this will include coordinating procedures with other surgeons to limit repetitive anesthesia when possible.

Bedside Versus Operative Debridement

Large or complex wounds can be devastating injuries for older adults, with a similar impact on quality of life, morbidity, and mortality as a proximal femur fracture. In fact, in frail institutionalized older adults, the 2 may be present concurrently and may be a symptom of the overall frail status of the patient nearing end of life.[27] Even in the outpatient setting frailty is more common in older adults (age >70 years) being treated for wounds (75%) than in the general community (26%).[9,28] When the wound is related to a fall or immobility, particularly in patients manifesting one or more element of frailty, a holistic discussion with the entire team, including the patient, the patient's significant others and the medical team is paramount. Determining whether a wound is likely to heal and the amount of pain and suffering that the patient is experiencing will depend on the wound etiology, medical comorbidities, and the duration and size of the wound. Assessment of the wound in conjunction with a global health assessment may lead the team to agree that a palliative approach is in the patient's best interest. In this case, topical wound care that emphasizes pain and odor reduction, prevention of infection, and moisture control are adopted. Many wounds improve with this nonoperative approach (**Box 1**). If it is determined that excisional debridement of the wound is the optimal treatment to facilitate healing or simplify

---

Box 1
Patient scenario 1

An 81-year-old woman survived a major and very complex surgery due to ischemic bowel with the input of multiple surgical disciplines, including thoracic, vascular, and general surgeons. During her recovery, she developed a pressure ulcer that has now become necrotic. Compared with her presurgical status she has had a marked decline in health. She is intermittently lucid. She has not previously discussed her treatment preferences with her family. Is surgery on the wound going to change the course of the patient's life, change management of the wound, and improve quality of life? Moreover, most importantly, is it possible to determine what Matters Most to this patient? How aggressive should the medical team be if the patient is readmitted to the hospital for concerns about a wound infection?

the wound care, the next step in shared decision-making is whether operative debridement would be more beneficial than bedside debridement.

Factors to consider for bedside debridement include whether the site of the wound is sensate, and if so, the degree of pain associated with the wound, the size and depth of the wound, whether the patient is anticoagulated, the ability to optimally position for access to the wound, and the urgency of debridement, particularly with obviously infected wounds. Bedside debridement may be a temporizing measure until the patient can be medically optimized to safely undergo anesthesia or may be a way to further assess the wound before elective operative debridement. However, serial bedside debridement either may be sufficient to promote wound healing or may be used in conjunction with topical debriding agents or negative pressure wound therapy with or without instillation.[29] The advantages of operative debridement include the ability to administer anesthesia and analgesia, improved access to deeper tissues, ability to obtain hemostasis, and better eradication of deep-seated infection with optimized tissue biopsies, including bone if indicated. Another advantage may the opportunity to improve access to the wound bed by eliminating undermining and tunneling, thereby reducing pain during subsequent dressing changes. Disadvantages include the previously outlined impact of anesthesia on mentation, as well as the potential for hemodynamic changes in patients with complex comorbid illnesses. As tissue evolves over time, a single debridement may not be sufficient and the patient and caregivers should be apprised of this (**Box 2**).

Diagnosis and Mixed Disease

As people age, they accumulate comorbidities, including venous insufficiency, arterial insufficiency, diabetes, and congestive heart failure with leg edema. These conditions make diagnosis and treatment more difficult and misdiagnosis can lead to delayed treatment. Many patients present with ulcerations on their lower extremities that they may attribute to trauma or that may have been diagnosed as a venous ulcer. It is important to maintain a high index of suspicion for alternative diagnoses when an ulcer does not heal when treated with the usual standard of care and consider a biopsy. This may be done at the bedside with a small wedge excision or punch biopsy that includes a portion of normal adjacent skin.[30] If a diagnosis of malignancy is relatively certain, based on the experience of the clinician, a history of significant sun exposure and skin quality that is characteristic of sun damage, proceeding directly to excisional biopsy is a reasonable option and is both diagnostic and therapeutic.

Box 2
Patient scenario 2

An 88-year-old man presented to the hospital after his neighbors noticed that they had not seen him for several days. Initial evaluation revealed altered mental status, dehydration, acute kidney injury, rhabdomyolysis, and deep tissue injuries on the right arm, hip, and heel. He was diagnosed with a urinary tract infection, started on antibiotics and a wound consult was placed. Increasingly patients are presenting to the hospital after being "found down" at home. Older adults who live alone may develop severe pressure injuries after falling and being unable to get up. These "incidental" pressure injuries usually begin as a deep tissue injury and will evolve over time. In these cases, there is no urgency to debride the wound but close follow-up is required as the patient recovers from the inciting event and is left with a high-grade pressure injury. This allows time to involve the patient and the entire care team in developing a plan of care that meets the needs and wishes of the patient.

Almost all pretibial lesions require skin grafting because there is minimal soft tissue laxity and closing these wounds under tension nearly always results in dehiscence.

Flaps and Grafts in Older Adults

An early and aggressive approach to wound closure reduces cost, improves quality of life, and prevents readmission to the hospital. Thus, once a wound has been optimized by debridement and topical wound care, it may be prudent to provide definitive coverage. However, unless hardware is exposed, flap reconstruction, particularly for pressure ulcers is an elective procedure. Although there are no randomized controlled trials, small case series suggest that in selected cases, definitive coverage may be successfully accomplished in older adults.[31] Factors specific to the flap itself include the availability of well-vascularized local flaps, ability to immobilize the area postoperatively, assessment of whether the patient will be able to avoid pressure on the surgical site, and the pain associated with the surgical site. Additional factors include the comorbidities, duration and potential blood loss for the surgical procedure, nutritional status, smoking or alcohol use, and potential for an agreement to rehabilitation postoperatively. In some cases, the need for fecal and urinary diversion is also a consideration.

Grafting Techniques and Technology

Older adults with large open wounds or skin cancers are rarely offered skin grafts due to the belief that they will not heal and that the donor site is very painful. It has been reported that lower extremity skin grafts have a high failure rate, which is accentuated in older adults, yet this is the very population that requires rapid healing after skin cancer excision or treatment of traumatic skin tears and avulsions.[23,32] The most likely reason for graft failure is failure to treat the underlying comorbidities, particularly venous insufficiency. Due to the high prevalence in older adults, treatment of lower extremity trauma, hematomas, and skin cancers is often complicated by venous insufficiency. Both venous insufficiency and peripheral arterial disease need to be considered when evaluating a patient with a lower extremity wound. If edema is not managed postoperatively, the wounds will not heal. Similarly, depending on the location of the wound, revascularization may be required to ensure healing and should be considered either before excision and grafting or early after a traumatic injury.

In addition to graft healing, the donor site has been the source of concern, particularly related to pain.[33] In light of these concerns, this author undertook the development of a standardized protocol to produce consistent and reliable outcomes with minimal pain. A retrospective, Institutional Review Board approved observational cohort study of all patients aged 70 years and older undergoing split-thickness skin grafting of lower extremity wounds between 2017 and 2020 was performed. Eighteen patients with ages ranging from 73 to 97 years were included. The most common comorbidities were venous insufficiency, congestive heart failure, and diabetes. The wound sizes ranged from 6.25 to 234 cm^2. Fourteen of the 18 patients were treated with multilayer compression wraps for edema control. Median time to healing of the graft was 35.5 days, median donor site time to healing was 20.7 days. Pain at the first clinic visit was minimal (median = 0, range = 0–8).[34] These results demonstrate that in the properly selected older adults, even large grafts and large donor sites heal rapidly and with minimal morbidity. In this study and in the author's experience, many of these wounds require specialty care that is beyond the scope of what most primary care offices are equipped to provide. Comprehensive wound care centers that provide a multidisciplinary approach with specialized nursing care, advanced wound care products, and close collaboration with the surgeon are critical for successful outcomes.

Innovations

The most complex patients may benefit from innovations in surgical technique and alternatives to the usual split-thickness skin graft or flap reconstruction. Fortunately, advances in wound care have led to several innovations that can promote rapid healing and preserve tissue. Hydrosurgical debridement is one technique that can be used to tangentially debride the surface, reduce irregular contours, and prepare the wound bed for grafting with less tissue and blood loss than conventional scalpel debridement.[35] After debridement, patients with very large wounds may benefit from a 2-stage approach in which a temporizing matrix is applied to reduce insensible water loss, reduce inflammation, and reduce the intensity and frequency of wound care. By covering the wound immediately after debridement, pain and inflammation are reduced, which allows less use of opioid analgesics. This is especially valuable for patients with necrotizing soft tissue infections or large pressure or avulsion injuries with extensive tissue loss after a fall. This first stage allows the patient to be stabilized, medically optimized and promotes edema reduction in preparation for definitive reconstruction. These advanced products become integrated into the patient's own tissue and promote the formation of a neodermis. The combination with negative pressure wound therapy aids in edema reduction and keeping the matrix in place in mobile areas.

Autologous tissue is recognized as optimal for providing definitive closure, yet for older adults with multiple medical problems, creating a large wound to close an injury can be problematic. New innovations that expand autologous skin to cover a large surface area are extremely advantageous. Micrografting was originally developed in the 1950s but further refinements in processing and delivery can provide expansion of thin split-thickness grafts in ratios up to 100:1.[36] Originally developed for burn wounds, "spray-on cells" are now available in the United States for use on multiple wound types.[37,38]

With this technique and delivery device, it is possible to harvest a very thin split-thickness skin graft (0.006–0.008 inches), enzymatically digest the tissue, and create a cell suspension that can be sprayed on the wound and the donor site to promote relatively rapid healing with good esthetic results. Although patient selection is critical due to the added expense of the device, this technology is particularly advantageous for older adults, with preexisting comorbidities that will delay healing, who sustain large open wounds due to avulsion injuries, hematomas, or infection (**Fig. 1**).

Postoperative Care

Safe and consistent postoperative care of older adults undergoing surgery for their wounds can make the difference between outpatient care with rapid healing and development of complications with need for multiple hospital admissions. Priorities include pain management, edema control, and mobility.

Many physicians are reluctant to aggressively treat pain in older adults, and the patients may be reluctant to use opioid analgesics due to fear of addiction. However, adequate pain control can optimize healing by reducing vasoconstriction and allow for adequate wound care with cleansing of the operative site. A good rule of thumb is to "go low and slow," by treating initially with nonopioid analgesics, and titrating in low-dose opioids as needed, primarily for dressing changes and to allow adequate nocturnal pain control while avoiding oversedation and opioid-induced apnea.

Nearly all older adults have some degree of lower extremity edema that will be exacerbated by the inflammation from an injury or surgical procedure, as well as from postoperative fluid shifts. Thus, after any procedure on the lower extremity, including

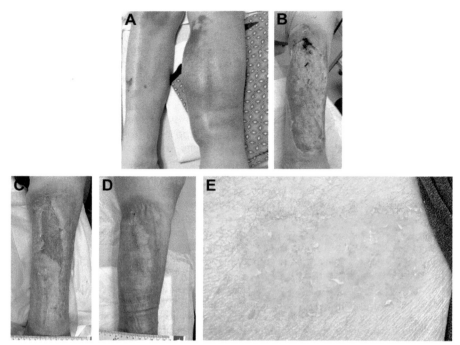

Fig. 1. (*A*) A 72-year-old woman, end-stage renal disease on hemodialysis, h/o calciphylaxis, hit her leg on the edge of a bed. Developed large expanding hematoma due to low platelet count. Unable to salvage overlying skin. (*B*) Topical treatment of the wound until ready to graft. Initial size was 262 cm^2. (*C*) RECELL was used to minimize donor site. Postoperative week 7: the wound measured 35 cm^2. (*D*) Complete healing at 11 weeks. (*E*) Donor site measured 2 × 4 cm^2. Healed in 13 days with no pain reported.

excision and closure of a skin lesion, debridement or skin grafting, compression should be applied. The type of compression must be based on the assessment of adequate lower extremity perfusion but even light compression and elevation will prevent excessive edema and optimize results.

Older adults consider impaired physical function to be an unacceptable outcome of medical treatment. Unfortunately, the geriatric-specific risk factors that lead to postoperative functional decline correlate closely with the reason that patients require wound-related surgery, including history of falls, malnutrition, use of mobility aids, and cognitive decline.[39] The deleterious effects of prolonged bedrest are well known; however, it is worth emphasizing that substantial muscle atrophy occurs within 72 hours of bedrest and that this effect is much more profound in the older adult.[40,41] Thus, rapid postoperative mobilization is critical to obtaining good surgical outcomes.

Mobility aids, if not already in use, should be considered to facilitate rapid and safe mobilization. If possible, this should be ascertained preoperatively so that the older adult can practice and get comfortable with the aid. As noted previously, prehabilitation can be an important intervention to optimize postoperative outcomes, especially mobility with or without a mobility aid and even in-bed mobility. However, most surgeries for wounds that would lead to impaired mobility are not elective. In these cases, postoperative physical therapy and occupational therapy, even if this requires a period of short-term inpatient rehabilitation, can help the older adult return and remain at home.

It is important to consider the impact of devices that are often used to facilitate wound healing on the lifestyle and mobility of the older adult. Specifically, tubing from drains and negative pressure wound therapy may become entangled, limit mobility, and can even become a tripping hazard. If critical to the surgical outcome, these tubes can be secured, or tubing shortened to reduce the risk of tripping or entanglement. Device noise and simply being connected to the negative pressure wound therapy device have also been cited as factors leading sleep deprivation, which can increase postoperative delirium.[42]

Approximately 50% of adults aged older than 80 years have nocturia resulting in voiding 2 times per night. There is some evidence suggesting that there is an increase in risk of falls and fractures in older adults with nocturia.[43] Although it has not been studied, it makes sense that when combined with reduced agility after a surgical procedure and/or pain from a wound, the potential for falls or nocturnal incontinence would be high. Thus, for the short term, one strategy is to provide male patients with a urinal or external catheter. External diversion is also available for women, although that requires a suction pump that would require insurance preauthorization. Another solution is to manage nocturnal incontinence with absorbent pads. The resulting skin maceration would not be acceptable for healing pelvic or proximal thigh wounds, flaps, or grafts, and therefore, an indwelling catheter may be required until the site is healed.

SUMMARY

From the foregoing, it should be clear that the surgical treatment of wounds in older adults requires a team approach that encompasses the patient, caregivers, ancillary care givers, and medical team. Basic principles of wound healing, including debridement, moisture management, reduction of contamination and optimizing tissue perfusion are imperative but there are other considerations specific to the older adult that need to be considered to achieve optimal outcomes. An in-depth conversation with the patient and their caregivers that outlines the planned surgical procedure, the anticipated postoperative care, the risks of postoperative function decline and the potential for delayed healing requiring frequent postoperative visits with close supervision are all details that need to be incorporated into shared decision-making.

CLINICS CARE POINTS

- Applying the principles of the 4 Ms and the GSV Program is critical in the overall surgical treatment of wounds in older adults.
- Wound debridement may be performed at the bedside or in the operating room depending on the complexity of the wound and the needs and wishes of the patient.
- Skin grafts can be performed safely with minimal morbidity in older adults with large open wounds.
- A team approach is required to optimize surgical treatment of older adults.

DISCLOSURE

The author has received no funding and declares no conflicts of interest associated with this article.

REFERENCES

1. Gould L, Abadir P, Brem H, et al. Chronic wound repair and healing in older adults: current status and future research. J Am Geriatr Soc 2015;63(3):427–38.
2. Alam W, Hasson J, Reed M. Clinical approach to chronic wound management in older adults. J Am Geriatr Soc 2021;69:1–8.
3. Berian JR, Rosenthal RA, Baker TL, et al. Hospital standards to promote optimal surgical care of the older adult: a report from the Coalition for Quality in Geriatric Surgery. Ann Surg 2018;267(2):280–90.
4. Gould LJ, Abadir PM, White-Chu F. Age, frailty, and impaired wound healing. In: *Principles and practice of geriatric surgery*. Cham, Switzerland: Springer; 2020. p. 465–82.
5. Hamel MB, Henderson WG, Khuri SF, et al. Surgical outcomes for patients aged 80 and older: morbidity and mortality from major noncardiac surgery. J Am Geriatr Soc 2005;53(3):424–9.
6. Lesser S, Zakharkin S, Louie C, et al. Clinician knowledge and behaviors related to the 4Ms framework of Age-Friendly Health Systems. J Am Geriatr Soc 2022; 70(3):789–800.
7. Carter MJ, DaVanzo J, Haught R, et al. Chronic wound prevalence and the associated cost of treatment in Medicare beneficiaries: changes between 2014 and 2019. J Med Econ 2023;26(1):894–901.
8. Correˆa NF, de Brito MJ, de Carvalho Resende MM, et al. Impact of surgical wound dehiscence on health-related quality of life and mental health. J Wound Care 2016;25(10):561–70.
9. Espaulella-Ferrer M, Espaulella-Panicot J, Noell-Boix R, et al. Assessment of frailty in elderly patients attending a multidisciplinary wound care centre: a cohort study. BMC Geriatr 2021;21(1):727.
10. Guest JF, Fuller GW, Vowden P. Cohort study evaluating the burden of wounds to the UK's National Health Service in 2017/2018: update from 2012/2013. BMJ Open 2020;10(12):e045253.
11. Horn SD, Fife CE, Smout RJ, et al. Wound healing index for chronic wounds. Wound Repair Regen 2013;21:823–32.
12. Eckert KA, Fife CE, Carter MJ. The impact of underlying conditions on quality-of-life measurement among patients with chronic wounds, as measured by utility values: a review with an additional study. Adv Wound Care 2023;12(12):680–95.
13. Chimukangara M, Helm MC, Frelich MJ, et al. A 5-item frailty index based on NSQIP data correlates with outcomes following paraesophageal hernia repair. Surg Endosc 2017;31(6):2509–19.
14. McGovern J, Grayston A, Coates D, et al. The relationship between the modified frailty index score (mFI-5), malnutrition, body composition, systemic inflammation and short-term clinical outcomes in patients undergoing surgery for colorectal cancer. BMC Geriatr 2023;23:9.
15. Ma M, Peters XD, Zhang LM, et al. Multisite Implementation of an American College of surgeons geriatric surgery quality Improvement initiative. J Am Coll Surg 2023;237(2):171–81.
16. Mate K, Fulmer T, Pelton L, et al. Evidence for the 4Ms: interactions and outcomes across the care Continuum. J Aging Health 2021;33(7–8):469–81.
17. Swanson T, Ousey K, Haesler E, et al. IWII wound infection in clinical practice consensus document: 2022 update. J Wound Care 2022;31(Sup12):S10–21.

18. Kapoor P, Chen L, Saripella A, et al. Prevalence of preoperative cognitive impairment in older surgical patients: a systematic review and meta-analysis. J Clin Anesth 2022;76:110574.
19. Fick DM, Steis MR, Waller JL, et al. Delirium superimposed on dementia is associated with prolonged length of stay and poor outcomes in hospitalized older adults. J Hosp Med 2013;8(9):500–5.
20. Peters X, Matlic M, Robinson TN, et al. Cognitive screening in older patients may help optimize outcomes. ACS Bull 2023;108(9):11–5.
21. Hartley P, Keating JL, Jeffs KJ, et al. Exercise for acutely hospitalized older medical patients. Cochrane Database Syst Rev 2022;11:CD005955. Accessed 09 November 2023.
22. Strong for Surgery: Prehabilitation. The American College of Surgeons Web site. Available at: https://https://www.facs.org/for-patients/strong-for-surgery/prehabilitation/. Accessed November 9, 2023.
23. Martínez-Velilla N, Casas-Herrero A, Zambom-Ferraresi F, et al. Effect of exercise intervention on functional decline in very elderly patients during acute hospitalization: a randomized clinical trial. JAMA Intern Med 2019;179(1):28–36.
24. Cardoso R, Parola V, Neves H, et al. Physical rehabilitation Programs for Bedridden patients with prolonged immobility: a scoping review. Int J Environ Res Public Health 2022;19(11):6420.
25. Staheli B. and Rondeau B., Anesthetic considerations in the geriatric population, In: StatPearls [Internet]. Treasure Island (FL): StatPearls Publishing; 2023. Available at: https://pubmed.ncbi.nlm.nih.gov/34283503/. Accessed October 28, 2023.
26. Silva AR, Regueira P, Albuquerque E, et al. Estimates of geriatric delirium frequency in noncardiac surgeries and its evaluation across the Years: a systematic review and meta-analysis. J Am Med Dir Assoc 2021;22(3):613–20.e9.
27. Loggers SAI, Willems HC, Van Balen R, et al. Evaluation of quality of life after Nonoperative or operative management of proximal Femoral fractures in frail institutionalized patients: the FRAIL-HIP study. JAMA Surg 2022;157(5):424–34.
28. Rivas-Ruiz F, Mach n M, Contreras-Fernndez E, et al. Prevalence of frailty among community-dwelling elderly persons in Spain and factors associated with it. Eur J Gen Pract 2019;25:190–6.
29. Matiasek J, Djedovic G, Kiehlmann M, et al. Negative pressure wound therapy with instillation: effects on healing of category 4 pressure ulcers. Plast Aesthet Res 2018;5:36.
30. Alavi A, Niakosari F, Sibbald R. When and How to Perform a biopsy on a chronic wound. Adv Skin Wound Care 2010;23:132–40.
31. Lauer H, Goertz O, Kolbenschlag J, et al. Gluteal propeller flaps - a reliable reconstructive alternative for elderly patients with pressure ulcers of the sacrum. J Tissue Viability 2019;28(4):227–30.
32. Reddy S., El-Haddawi F., Fancourt M., et al., The incidence and risk factors for lower limb skin graft failure, *Dermatol Res Pract*, 2014, 582080, Available at: https://www.ncbi.nlm.nih.gov/pmc/articles/PMC4123529/. Accessed October 15, 2023.
33. Asuku M, Tzy-Chyi Y, Qi Y, et al. Split-thickness skin graft donor-site morbidity: a systematic literature review. Burns 2021;47(7):1525–46.
34. Gould LJ. (2022, April 6-10) A Skin Graft Protocol to Heal Lower Extremity Wounds in Older Adults: Success through Collaboration. Conference presentation abstract, Symposium on Advanced Wound Care Spring, April 6-10 2022, Phoenix, AZ.

35. Liu J, Ko JH, Secretov E, et al. Comparing the hydrosurgery system to conventional debridement techniques for the treatment of delayed healing wounds: a prospective, randomised clinical trial to investigate clinical efficacy and cost-effectiveness. Int Wound J 2015;12(4):456–61.
36. Biswas A, Bharara M, Hurst C, et al. The micrograft concept for wound healing: strategies and applications. J Diabetes Sci Technol 2010;4(4):808–19.
37. Holmes JH. A Brief history of RECELL and its current indications. J Burn Care Res 2022;44(S1):S48–9.
38. RECELL Autologous Cell Harvesting Device.US Food and Drug Administration web site. Available at: https://www.fda.gov/vaccines-blood-biologics/approved-blood-products/recell-autologous-cell-harvesting-device. Published 2023.Accessed November 1, 2023.
39. Zhang LM, Hornor MA, Robinson T, et al. Evaluation of postoperative functional health status decline among older adults. JAMA Surg 2020;155(10):950–8.
40. Guedes LPCM, De Oliveira MLC, Carvalho GDA. Deleterious effects of prolonged bed rest on the body systems of the elderly. Rev Bras Geriatr Gerontol 2018;21:499–506.
41. Dronkers J, Witteman B, van Meeteren N. Surgery and functional mobility: doing the right thing at the right time. Tech Coloproctol 2016;20:339–41.
42. Miyanaga A, Miyanaga T, Sakai K, et al. Patient experience of negative pressure wound therapy: a qualitative study. Nurs Open 2023;10(3):1415–25.
43. Pesonen JS, Vernooij RWM, Cartwright R, et al. The impact of nocturia on falls and fractures: a systematic review and meta-analysis. J Urology 2020;201:674–83.

Infectious Aspects of Chronic Wounds

Natalie E. Nierenberg, MD, MPH[a],
Jeffrey M. Levine, MD, AGSF, CWS-P[b],*

KEYWORDS

- Skin and soft tissue infections (SSTI) • Pressure injury • Necrotizing infection
- Biofilm • Osteomyelitis • Cutaneous candidiasis • Sepsis • Cellulitis

KEY POINTS

- Geriatric patients can have an atypical or muted presentation for infection in an acute, subacute, and/or chronic wounds.
- The clinical spectrum of skin infections is highly variable and ranges from mild infections to life-threatening diseases.
- Since 2000, in patients more than the age of 65 years, the incidence of skin and soft tissue infections (SSTIs) has doubled and currently accounts for nearly half of Emergency Department visits, which is very costly to the health care system.
- The new definition of acute bacterial skin and skin structure infections (ABSSSI) was designed to allow homogeneity in patients included in clinical trials. However, important ABSSSI disease entities are excluded from this definition, and FDA guidance does not address the most common of these infections in geriatric patients and patients with diabetes including: animal or human bites, necrotizing fasciitis, diabetic foot infection, pressure injury infection, myonecrosis, and ecthyma gangrenosum.
- The microbial composition within the surface biofilm of a wound does not always correlate with the pathogens responsible for the tissue infection. When and how to culture the appropriate part of the skin or soft tissue is essential for proper care.

SPECIAL CONSIDERATIONS FOR GERIATRIC PATIENTS WITH CHRONIC WOUNDS

Geriatric patients have unique considerations that influence how infections present clinically. Management of infections is very challenging in the elderly due to multiple comorbidities, changes in drug pharmacokinetics and pharmacodynamics, and the presence of polypharmacy with the inherent risk of adverse drug reactions and drug–drug or drug–disease interactions.[1]

[a] Wound Care, Department of Infectious Diseases, Tufts Medical Center, Boston, MA 02111, USA; [b] Icahn School of Medicine at Mount Sinai, New York, NY 10010, USA
* Corresponding author.
E-mail address: jlevinemd@shcny.com

Clin Geriatr Med 40 (2024) 471–480
https://doi.org/10.1016/j.cger.2024.03.001
0749-0690/24/© 2024 Elsevier Inc. All rights reserved.

geriatric.theclinics.com

Since 2000, in patients older than 65 years, the incidence of skin and soft tissue infections (SSTIs) has doubled and currently accounts for nearly half of Emergency Department visits.[2] The clinical spectrum of skin infections is highly variable and ranges from mild infections to life-threatening diseases.[3] The new definition of acute bacterial skin and skin structure infections (ABSSSI) was designed to allow homogeneity in patients included in clinical trials. However, important ABSSSI disease entities are excluded from this definition and FDA guidance does not address infections needing more complex treatment regimens, including animal or human bites, necrotizing fasciitis, diabetic foot infection, pressure injury infection, myonecrosis, and ecthyma gangrenosum.[4] Many of these excluded, more complex, or atypical SSTI disease entities are frequent in the elderly. Moreover, the older patients are usually excluded from randomized controlled trials. Therefore, use caution when applying results of ABSSSI clinical trials to patients >65 years of age with necrotizing fasciitis, diabetic foot infection, pressure injury infection, and/or other complex or atypical SSTI.[5]

Infection interferes with several steps in the wound-healing pathway.[6] Inflammatory mediators produced by bacteria inhibit wound healing and cause cell death. Necrotic tissue prevents new tissue growth because it is physically occupying the healthy tissue space, and it is a substrate for for bacterial proliferation. Foreign bodies within a wound are a sanctuary for ongoing infection. They can present as a draining sinus or abscess around ingrown hair or stitch abscess from nonabsorbable sutures, infected surgical mesh, retained bullet, and hardware infection. For the wounds to heal, the foreign bodies should be removed or the infection suppressed with chronic antibiotics.

Ischemia is a condition that results in chronic nonhealing wounds and can be seen in arterial insufficiency, venous hypertension, and pressure injuries. In patients with arterial insufficiency, arterial blood flow to the tissue is diminished, leading to a decrease in the delivery of oxygen and nutrients to the wound, and an impairment in the removal of metabolic waste products from the wound. Limb-threatening ischemia develops when blood flow to the extremity is insufficient to meet the metabolic demands of the tissue, manifesting as rest pain or nonhealing wounds. Due to the chronic deficiency of oxygen and nutrients, the skin of the affected limb is not able to maintain normal tissue architecture. Clinically, this is manifested as a shiny skin surface with a paucity of hair. The metabolic demands to maintain intact skin are higher than the metabolic demands to heal a wound. A simple cut or abrasion on the skin caused by poor fitting shoes can alter the balance of metabolic demand, leading to a chronic wound. The most common cause of arterial insufficiency ulcers is the obstruction of large and medium-size arteries, which causes atherosclerosis. Other conditions that affect small arteries such as vasculitis, thromboangiitis obliterans, and scleroderma can also cause ischemic ulcers as well as certain viral infections.

In patients with chronic deep vein thrombosis, arteriovenous fistula, or venous insufficiency, hydrostatic pressure is built up in the venous system, leading to venous hypertension in the setting of chronic deep vein thrombosis. This results in a loss of pressure gradient between the arterioles and the venules, leading to a slowing of the movement of blood within the capillaries. This sluggish movement of blood results in the sequestration of erythrocytes and leukocytes within the capillaries. Increased hydrostatic pressure within the capillaries results in capillary leak. The fibrinogen leaked from the capillaries of the dermis to form a fibrin cuff, which resulted in decreased oxygen permeability leading to tissue hypoxia and impaired wound healing. The leukocytes trapped in the capillaries adhere to the endothelium and release inflammatory mediators and reactive oxygen metabolites. These in turn cause endothelial damage, obliteration of capillaries, and subsequent tissue ischemia. Capillaries of patients with venous stasis are also occluded by microthrombi that, in turn, reduce oxygen and nutrition to the tissue, predisposing to ulcer formation.

Pressure is a major factor in local ischemic injury. When the pressure applied to the skin is in excess of arteriolar pressure, tissue hypoxia and accumulation of waste products and free radicals occur, impeding healing and delivery of antibiotics and other medications to that tissue area. Tissues also vary in their susceptibility to pressure injuries. For soft tissue, muscle is the most susceptible, followed by subcutaneous fat, and then dermis. For this reason, extensive tissue damage can occur with little evidence of superficial injury. Differentiating pressure from infection and the combination of the two can be clinically challenging, especially when deeper tissues are involved. It requires a combination of all available tools and art of medicine in determining if and when systemic antibiotics are required and other modalities to excise infection.

Moisture from diaphoresis, urine, stool, gastric acid leaking from a tube, secretions from a tracheostomy site, or any other drainage of bodily fluid on the skin's surface is damaging and increases the risk for infection because the skin is broken down by the acids and other proteins in the secretions. Once there is a break in the skin's protective surface, which is much more vulnerable in older people, then the microbes that colonize the skin's surface can penetrate the deeper tissues and create infection. This infection can be rapidly progressive in the form of necrotizing cellulitis and bacteria can invade implanted medical devices and set up biofilm that is nearly impossible to eradicate without explant of the device. From an infection standpoint, moisture management is extremely important to prevent invasive infection. Cracks in dry skin present similar risks for invasive infection.

STRUCTURAL AND FUNCTIONAL CHANGES IN AGED SKIN THAT INCREASE THE RISK OF INFECTION

Skin aging is a complex process influenced by intrinsic (chronologic skin aging; genetic) and extrinsic (photoaging; environmental) factors that affect the structure and function of the epidermis and dermis.[7] These changes reduce the ability of skin cells to proliferate with eventual progression to senescence. There is epidermal atrophy and fibroblast senescence as well as decreased synthesis and accelerated breakdown of dermal collagen fibers. Altered fibroblast production affects skin healing by dermal atrophy and delayed collagen synthesis. Skin aging is a health risk because, with more skin fragility and impaired wound healing, there is an increased incidence of infection and malignancy.

Reduced inflammatory response, altered melanocyte function, reduced vitamin D production, reduced sensory function, thinning of the adipose layer, decreased estrogen, and altered pH with aging decrease skin integrity and increase infection. Similar physiologic changes are relevant in diabetics along with other critical changes. Particularly relevant to infection risk in diabetics and with aging is (1) alterations in skin pH and (2) reduced sensory function.

Alterations in skin pH are mediated by the skin microbiome, which is critical to understanding the increased risk of skin infection as we age and with chronic, immunosuppressive diseases such as diabetes.[8] Akin to the human gut microbiome being a map of all of the microorganisms that live within and interact with gut cells to dictate gut and other organ health, the skin microbiome is the diverse ecosystem of microorganisms that naturally reside within our skin. Each square centimeter of skin has up to one million microbes (bacteria, viruses, and fungi). The skin microbiome composition is affected by intrinsic and extrinsic factors. Just as oral antibiotics alter the gut microbiome, topical antimicrobials as well as various wavelengths of light affect the skin microbiome.

Imbalances of the skin microbiota, an essential element of the skin barrier system, can increase the risk of infection.[9] Moreover, 16S PCR studies have demonstrated that with aging, there is a higher diversity of the microbes comprising the skin microbiome. Higher diversity may indicate increased susceptibility to pathogenic invasion and infection with a reduced quantity of protective organisms, an increased abundance of less protective species, and an increase in the variety of organisms that are more pathogenic.

METABOLIC CONDITIONS

Several metabolic conditions contribute to the development of infected nonhealing wounds.

Diabetes Mellitus

There are several factors related to diabetes that contribute to the pathogenesis of diabetic foot ulcers. Damage to the sensory, motor, and autonomic nerve fibers affects peripheral sensation, motor innervation of small muscles in the foot, and fine vasomotor control of the pedal circulation. The loss of protective sensation leads to the lack of awareness of sustained pressure on the tissue or injury to the tissue. Motor neuropathy usually affects the innervation of the small intrinsic muscles of the feet, resulting in the unopposed action of the larger muscles in the anterior tibial compartment. This leads to the subluxation of the proximal metatarsal-phalangeal joints, giving the feet the appearance of claw toes. Consequently, the pressure is redistributed abnormally to the metatarsal heads, whereby the reactive thickening of the skin (callus) forms. Ischemic necrosis of the tissue under the callused skin eventually leads to the breakdown of the skin, resulting in a neuropathic ulcer with the typical punched-out appearance.

Autonomic neuropathy is characterized by a lack of autonomic tone in the arteriolar and capillary circulation, causing the shunting of blood from the arterioles directly to the veins, thus bypassing the tissue that needs the nutrients.[10] Although the feet may have bounding pulses and distended veins, the tissue may lack the perfusion needed for healing and to fight infection. Additionally, the loss of autonomic innervation to the sweat glands of the feet results in dry, scaly skin that can crack easily, allowing bacteria to penetrate.

The Charcot foot is a late complication of diabetes and is characterized by the collapse of the arch of the midfoot.[11] Osteopenia due to the arteriolar-venous shunting of autonomic neuropathy combined with small intrinsic muscle wasting, lead to the loss of structural integrity of the bone. Stress and minor trauma induce fracture of weakened bone, putting more stress on the adjacent weakened bones, and the cycle repeats, ultimately leading to gross deformity. The resulting abnormal bony prominences that form greatly increase the risk of ulceration.

Diabetes also affects microvascular beds by altering the structure of the basement membrane, the integrity of the capillary wall, the regulatory function of the endothelium, and the propensity for microvascular macrovascular disease in diabetes, resulting in tissue ischemia and impaired wound healing.

Malnutrition

Malnutrition is associated with an increased risk of wound infection, which has deleterious effects on wound healing.[12] Fatty acids are essential for the inflammatory phase of wound healing as they provide the arachidonic acid substrate for eicosanoid synthesis. Proteins are required for the proliferation of fibroblasts and the synthesis and deposition of collagen. Proteins are also required for important immunologic functions such as the phagocytic activity of macrophages, T-cell function, and complement and antibody production. Malnutrition can impair wound healing by prolonging the inflammatory phase and by reducing the proliferation of fibroblasts and the deposition of collagen.

Immunosuppression

Systemic immunosuppression can contribute to the development of nonhealing wounds.[13] Corticosteroids interfere with all major steps of the wound-healing process in both animal and human studies. In the inflammatory phase, corticosteroids decrease the expression of cytokines that are responsible for the recruitment of inflammatory cells, as well as the expression of adhesion molecules responsible for the adhesion and migration of granulocytes. In the proliferative phase, corticosteroids reduce the levels of transforming growth factor and keratinocyte growth factor, which attenuates fibroblast proliferation and wound epithelialization. In the remodeling phase, corticosteroids impair collagen accumulation as well as collagen turnover.

Clinically, patients who are on chronic corticosteroids that undergo surgery have a significantly increased infection rate as well as dehiscence rate. Immunosuppressive agents can suppress the expression of inflammatory mediators that are involved in the wound-healing process. Immunosuppressive agents inhibit the proliferation of immune cells and may blunt the inflammatory phase of wound healing. Chemotherapeutic agents, particularly those that target vascular endothelial growth factor (VEGF) and epidermal growth factor receptor (EGFR), can have detrimental effects on wound healing. Inhibition of VEGF results in the suppression of angiogenesis, which is an important part of wound healing. Epidermal growth factor receptor inhibitors can negatively impact wound healing by inhibiting epithelialization.

Radiation

Radiation therapy used in the treatment of cancer can cause subclinical radiation dermatitis that delays wound healing and sometimes results in chronic nonhealing wounds. Ionizing radiation causes cellular damage by breaking the double-stranded cellular DNA and releasing free radicals resulting in apoptosis and cellular necrosis. Radiation therapy also causes eccentric myointimal proliferation in the small arteries and arterioles, which may cause luminal thrombosis and ischemia, which can progress to tissue necrosis.

DIAGNOSTIC CHALLENGE OF INFECTION

Determining if a wound is infected and if it requires systemic antimicrobial therapy in older, immunocompromised patients or those with diabetes is challenging. Diabetics are immunocompromised and any immunocompromised patient often have atypical presentation for infection in a chronic wound.[14] This means that wound assessment in a diabetic or geriatric patient requires special attention. The continuum of acute, subacute, and chronic infection is like a pendulum that swings back and forth over time, as other systemic and extrinsic factors change.[15] It helps to have continuity of care and observation of wound characteristics over time with photographic documentation. Management depends primarily on deciding if a wound is acutely infected and/or if there are new host factors inhibiting healing.

BIOBURDEN AND BIOFILM

Understanding the microbial milieu of a wound's biofilm is critical in understanding a wound's current state of activity. Biofilm can be thought of as the substrate or base of the wound. A clean base and elimination of biofilm leads to more rapid healing. Serial debridement to excise biofilm is a mainstay of treatment to get a nonhealing wound into the active healing phase. Persistence of biofilm is the primary reason an infected device will never be "cured" of infection.[16] These micromatrices of bacteria, fungi, and virus attach to the wound bed or foreign body and multiply by their innate reproductive cycle. Most systemic antimicrobials are ineffective in attacking microbes that are within a biofilm adhered to a foreign body.[17] They are also largely ineffective in disrupting the reproduction of microbes within a chronically infected open wound. This is why serial debridement is effective as it mechanically removes the microbial "buildup" or biofilm that rebuilds over time within a wound bed. Some biofilms are harder to mechanically remove than others. Without the removal of a device that has been exposed to microbes, that device and its surrounding soft tissue or bone will never be cured of infection.[18] This is the rationale for chronic suppressive therapy of hardware infections in scenarios whereby the hardware cannot be removed, which is often the case in older patients with cardiac and/or orthopedic hardware.

The biofilm microbial composition on an exposed wound bed does not always correlate with the pathogens responsible for a developing soft tissue cellulitis. It is not uncommon to culture the biofilm, then remove the biofilm and culture the underlying soft tissue and then have different organisms or the same organism with different antimicrobial susceptibility patterns.[19] Often the organisms in the biofilm are more drug-resistant than the organisms affecting the soft tissue beneath them.

THE INFECTIOUS CONTINUUM: CONTAMINATION, CELLULITIS, AND SEPSIS
Contamination

Contamination is the overgrowth of potentially pathogenic microbes at the wound's surface. The contaminated wound bed can easily be cleansed with the application of topical cleansing solutions and antiseptics because the microbes have not yet replicated sufficiently to invade the surrounding tissue and/or evade host defenses. If not adequately cleansed, these microbes will continue to replicate and form the biofilm or "slough" at the wound base.[20]

Never to take a swab culture of the surface of a wound for the purposes of determining empiric antimicrobial therapy. Instead, deep cultures obtained from the layer of tissue with blood supply is preferred. This sample more adequately indicates the causative organism/s in a chronic wound that invade and infect the surrounding soft tissue. The results of deeper tissue culture can more appropriately guide systemic therapy.

Cellulitis and Sepsis

Cellulitis is the infection of the skin and/or soft tissue. In the setting of a chronic wound, this would be the tissue adjacent to the wound itself. If the tissue surrounding the chronic wound is warm, red, painful, and/or there is progressive darkening, discoloration, desquamation or blistering, change in temperature, swelling, tenderness, change in the drainage, malodor, and/or other systemic signs of infection such as fevers, chills, sweats, decreased appetite, decreased energy, altered mental status or delirium, change in blood sugar control, change in WBC (higher or lower), or an increase in inflammatory markers (CRP or ESR), then cellulitis should be presumed and treated empirically after appropriate cultures have been obtained when feasible.[3]

Imaging with ultrasound, X-ray, CT, and/or MRI can be helpful to confirm a suspected diagnosis, and is especially important in other types of SSTIs, but should never replace the clinical examination. Radiographic imaging can lag up to two weeks from the clinical examination. Additionally, older patients and diabetics are immunocompromised, and examination findings can be subtle, and if not addressed in a timely manner can progress rapidly to sepsis with bacteremia or fungemia, or necrotizing infections.

Patients with dark skin require more careful physical examination and consideration as it may be more difficult to visualize erythema or other color changes associated with cellulitis and other soft tissue infections. Palpation of affected and adjacent skin and soft tissue to assess the temperature and pain and other indicators while using an adjunct light source to compare subtle discolorations from the adjacent soft tissue is critical to avoid missing the diagnosis in dark pigmented patients or patients with chronic venous stasis changes or brawny edema with chronic hyperpigmentation. Always listen to the patient and/or their caregivers and obtain their input to gather helpful clinical clues.

CUTANEOUS CANDIDIASIS

Yeast, most commonly *Candida* species, are ubiquitous in our environment and on our skin and our mucosal surfaces. Aberrations in skin and/or gut microbiota due to stress, acute illness, antimicrobial systemic therapy that depletes the healthy microbes that suppress *Candida* growth, permitting *Candida* overgrowth. Diabetes with increased blood sugar promotes *Candida* overgrowth, particularly in moist environments such as skin folds or in the acutely ill, diaphoretic, and/or incontinent patient.

Cutaneous candidiasis can also be thought of as a window into the overall health of a patient's skin and risk of SSTI, as candidiasis indicates a decrease in the protective barrier of the skin. Moisture management and protection of skin integrity are of the utmost importance in aging patients and those with diabetes as well those on broad-spectrum antibiotics or other risk factors mentioned above.[21] Candidemia can result from cutaneous candidiasis but this is less frequent than the candidiasis causing a break down in the skin which then allows pathogens such as MRSA, *Streptococcus*, and so forth to enter the soft tissue and the bloodstream causing bacteremia, sepsis and death.

NECROTIZING SOFT TISSUE INFECTIONS

Geriatric patients, diabetics, and immunocompromised patients can rapidly progress from contamination to critical colonization to mild surrounding cellulitis to cellulitis and/or abscess to necrotizing cellulitis and/or fasciitis.[22] These infections progress within hours crossing the fascial planes without regard for tissue boundaries. Whenever a patient's pain on examination is out of proportion to the visual clinical examination, suspect, prepare for and exclude a necrotizing infection.[23] With a skin marker, draw lines around the erythema, time and date stamp them. If any spread beyond the initial line within 15 minutes, notify surgery immediately. Obtain blood, urine and wound cultures when possible before starting empiric therapy but do not delay starting broad-spectrum Gram-negative, Gram-positive and anaerobic coverage with an antibiotic combination that may include clindamycin, vancomycin, and piperacillin/tazobactam or meropenem (depending on your hospital's antibiogram). Obtain plain films or CT imaging looking for gas in the soft tissue, but do not allow spreading erythema or spreading warmth or discoloration delay surgery notification and OR preparation.

Once in the OR, the surgeon should send deep tissue cultures for aerobic and anaerobic culture and tissue samples to pathology to look for signs of necrotizing infection. Most often the surgeon can determine if necrotizing infection is present based on the appearance, quality, and depth or extent of tissue destruction. Often there is a "dishwasher" dirty appearance to the fluid released with initial fasciotomy. Serial surgeries are often necessary until there is control of toxin-mediated tissue destruction.

OSTEOMYELITIS

Osteomyelitis may be caused by bacteria or fungi, and can be acute, subacute, or chronic. It can involve bone with hardware or bone that has been previously injured and hematogenously infected from bacteremia/fungemia or from seeding the bone from an adjacent open wound or invasion of bone from a nearby deep tissue infection, pressure injury infection or hardware infection. Acute osteomyelitis is easier to diagnose. There is typically associated pain localized over or within the affected bone. When ESR and CRP are more than 100 in the setting of acute bony pain or wound associated with the bone, this is usually diagnostic of acute osteomyelitis. Subacute and chronic osteomyelitis typically requires additional data including imaging and or bone biopsy with bone tissue sent to pathology and microbiology. MRI is the imaging modality preferred. WBC scans can occasionally be helpful when MRI is contraindicated.[24] If the bone is palpable within a diabetic foot ulcer and/or pressure injury that has other signs of infection, osteomyelitis can be assumed by "probe to bone" diagnosis.[25]

INFECTIONS INVOLVING HARDWARE

Establishing if implanted hardware is infected is not always straightforward, especially in geriatric patients and persons with diabetes. The presentation can be vague and consequently the diagnosis is often delayed. In any aged patient with altered mental status or delirium, infection should be excluded as a cause. It is optimal to obtain deep cultures from the device and/or tissue surrounding the device via aspiration, IR-guided sample, and/or OR collection of tissue adjacent to suspected infected hardware or a piece of the hardware itself.[26]

Once hardware infection has been established, options for source control are evaluated in consultation with the appropriate surgeon or surgical subspecialist (ie, if a ventricular assist device or mechanical heart valve, cardiothoracic surgery; if hip replacement, orthopedic surgery; if VP shunt, neurosurgery). If feasible, always remove the infected device. If the causative organism is *Staphylococcus aureus*, the recommendation is prompt device removal as these infections are difficult to cure and suppress. If the organism is a less virulent species, such as coagulase-negative *Staphylococcus* or a susceptible Gram-negative species, and hardware excision is high risk and/or the patient has high risk comorbidities for extraction, an acute systemic antibiotic regimen followed by chronic suppressive therapy can reasonably be offered.

CLINICS CARE POINTS: INFECTIOUS ASPECTS OF CHRONIC WOUNDS

- The primary care physician should always examine and document wounds, looking for changes that might indicate infection.
- Always have high level of suspicion for deep infection such as osteomyelitis, abscess, and necrotizing fasciitis, particularly in patients with diabetes.

- Metabolic and anatomic changes associated with aging skin increase the risk of infection.
- Surface wound swabs are not helpful for determining antimicrobial therapy. Deep tissue cultures are more appropriate to guide systemic therapy.
- Patients with dark skin require careful physical examination as it may be more difficult to visualize color changes associated with cellulitis and soft tissue infections.
- Osteomyelitis should always be suspected when wounds probe to bone. Diagnosis can be made with bone biopsy, MRI, or elevated CRP in the setting of bone pain.
- Advance directives should always be taken into account when constructing a treatment plan for infected wounds.

DISCLOSURE

The authors have nothing to disclose.

REFERENCES

1. Alam W, Hasson J, Reed M. Clinical approach to chronic wound management in older adults. J Am Geriatr Soc 2021;69(8):2327–34.
2. Kaye KS, Petty LA, Shorr AF, et al. Current epidemiology, etiology, and burden of acute skin infections in the United States. Clin Infect Dis 2019;68:S193–9.
3. Maher E, Anokhin A. Bacterial skin and soft tissue infections in older adults. Clin Geriatr Med 2024;40(1):117–30.
4. Itani KM, Shorr AF. FDA guidance for ABSSSI trials: implications for conducting and interpreting clinical trials. Clin Infect Dis 2014;58(Suppl 1):S4–9.
5. Falcone M, Tiseo G. Skin and soft tissue infections in the elderly. Curr Opin Infect Dis 2023;36(2):102–8.
6. Sandoz H. An overview of the prevention and management of wound infection. Nurs Stand 2022;37(10):75–82.
7. Levine JM. Clinical Aspects of aging skin: considerations for the wound care practitioner. Adv Skin Wound Care 2020;33(1):12–9.
8. Polk C, Sampson MM, Roshdy D, et al. Skin and soft tissue infections in patients with diabetes mellitus. Infect Dis Clin North Am 2021;35(1):183–97.
9. Shibagaki N, Suda W, Clavaud C, et al. Aging-related changes in the diversity of women's skin microbiomes associated with oral bacteria. Sci Rep 2017;7: 10567.
10. Freeman R. Autonomic peripheral neuropathy. Continuum (Minneap Minn) 2020; 26(1):58–71.
11. Trieb K. The Charcot foot: pathophysiology, diagnosis and classification. Bone Joint Lett J 2016;98-B(9):1155–9.
12. Stechmiller JK. Understanding the role of nutrition and wound healing. Nutr Clin Pract 2010;25(1):61–8.
13. Sorg H, Tilkorn DJ, Hager S, et al. Skin wound healing: an update on the current knowledge and concepts. Eur Surg Res 2017;58(1–2):81–94.
14. Bonham PA. Identifying and treating wound infection. J Gerontol Nurs 2009; 35(10):12–6.
15. van Duin D. Diagnostic challenges and opportunities in older adults with infectious diseases. Clin Infect Dis 2012;54:973–8.
16. Macià MD, Del Pozo JL, Díez-Aguilar M, et al. Microbiological diagnosis of biofilm-related infections. Enferm Infecc Microbiol Clín 2018;36(6):375–81. English, Spanish.

17. Rather MA, Gupta K, Mandal M. Microbial biofilm: formation, architecture, antibiotic resistance, and control strategies. Braz J Microbiol 2021;52(4):1701–18.
18. Khatoon Z, McTiernan CD, Suuronen EJ, et al. Bacterial biofilm formation on implantable devices and approaches to its treatment and prevention. Heliyon 2018;4(12):e01067. Available at: https://www.ncbi.nlm.nih.gov/pmc/articles/PMC 6312881/.
19. Venkatesan N, Perumal G, Doble M. Bacterial resistance in biofilm-associated bacteria. Future Microbiol 2015;10(11):1743–50.
20. Kingsley A. The wound infection continuum and its application to clinical practice. Ostomy/Wound Manag 2003;49(7A Suppl):1–7.
21. Taudorf EH, Jemec GBE, Hay RJ, et al. Cutaneous candidiasis - an evidence-based review of topical and systemic treatments to inform clinical practice. J Eur Acad Dermatol Venereol 2019;33(10):1863–73.
22. Stevens DL, Bryant AE. Necrotizing soft-tissue infections. N Engl J Med 2018; 378(10):971.
23. Madsen MB, Arnell P, Hyldegaard O. Necrotizing soft-tissue infections: clinical features and diagnostic aspects. Adv Exp Med Biol 2020;1294:39–52.
24. Palestro CJ. Radionuclide imaging of osteomyelitis. Semin Nucl Med 2015;45(1): 32–46.
25. Chicco M, Singh P, Beitverda Y, et al. Diagnosing pelvic osteomyelitis in patients with pressure ulcers: a systematic review comparing bone histology with alternative diagnostic modalities. J Bone Jt Infect 2020;6(1):21–32.
26. Dibartola AC, Swearingen MC, Granger JF, et al. Biofilms in orthopedic infections: a review of laboratory methods. APMIS 2017;125(4):418–28.

Nutritional Aspects of Wound Care

Nancy Munoz, DCN, MHA, RDN, FAND[a],*, Mary Litchford, PhD, RDN[b]

KEYWORDS

- Pressure injuries • Chronic wounds • Malnutrition • Nutrition • Wound care

KEY POINTS

- Sufficient nutrition is required for skin health and is essential for skin and tissue regeneration.
- Disease-related malnutrition concurrent with pressure injuries and disease-related wounds requires an interprofessional team to prioritize interventions for medical management of polymorbidities and nutrition interventions.
- Laboratory studies such as serum albumin, prealbumin, and other laboratory values may be useful in establishing the overall prognosis for the patient but are not considered sensitive indicators of nutritional status.

INTRODUCTION

Robust skin health and nutritional well-being are fundamental components of healthy living for all age groups.[1–3] Nutritional well-being depends on access to healthy foods and nutrition care services. Access to nutrient-dense foods is one of the social determinants of health in older adults.[4] Access to nutrition care is addressed in the International Declaration on the Human Right to Nutritional Care, supported by national clinical and medical societies.[5] While core components of nutritional well-being are recognized by medical communities worldwide, putting these concepts into practice to address malnutrition is yet to be fully achieved.

Malnutrition is a collective term that includes both undernutrition and malnutrition. It is due to deficiencies, excesses, and imbalances of macronutrients and micronutrients. Malnutrition presents with and without inflammation, is reported in underweight, normal weight, and overweight individuals, and is associated with undesirable alterations in body composition, and diminished functional status.[6–8] It is the leading cause of morbidity and mortality in older adults.[8] The Center for Disease Control and Prevention provisional data for 2018 to 2022 report that deaths from malnutrition in adults 65 years and older have more than doubled in 5 years.[9]

[a] Chief Nutrition and Food Service, VA Southern Nevada Healthcare System, Las Vegas, NV, USA; [b] Case Software, 5601 Forest Manor Drive, Greensboro, NC 27410, USA
* Corresponding author. 7041 Solana Ridge Drive, North Las Vegas, NV 89084.
E-mail address: Dr.NMunozRD@outlook.com

Clin Geriatr Med 40 (2024) 481–500
https://doi.org/10.1016/j.cger.2023.12.005
0749-0690/24/Published by Elsevier Inc.

geriatric.theclinics.com

The etiology of malnutrition is categorized as starvation-related malnutrition, chronic disease–related malnutrition (CDM), and acute disease–related malnutrition(ADM). Smith, 2022, reported that the prevalence of malnutrition in acute care was highest in older adults with CDM. In long-term care facilities, the prevalence of malnutrition is estimated to be more than 65% of residents.[10]

The burden of malnutrition falls on individuals, medical providers, and health care organizations in all care settings. Resources are available in both acute care and post-acute care settings to identify malnutrition, assess the quality of malnutrition care, and device tactics to increase reimbursement. The Malnutrition Quality Improvement Initiative (MQii) disseminates malnutrition standards of care in acute care settings (malnutritionquality.org). MQii spearheaded the development of the Global Malnutrition Composite Score (GMCS), an optional electronic clinical quality measure (eCQM) in the Hospital Inpatient Quality Reporting Program. Strategies to adopt GMCS as an eCQM are available at www.malnutritionquality.org.

In skilled nursing facilities (SNFs), the patient-driven payment model (PDPM) considers declining nutritional well-being and the risk for malnutrition on the Minimum Data Set (MDS) in determining reimbursement for residents in stays covered by Medicare Part A. PDPM to determine the comorbidity score replaced resource utilization groups in 2019. Key codings on the MDS associated with increased nontherapy ancillary costs are noted in **Table 1**. SNFs may receive higher reimbursement when a physician's diagnosis of malnutrition and/or morbid obesity is documented in the resident's health record and coded properly on the MDS (fee-for-service-payment/snfpps/pdpm" title="https://www.cms.gov/medicare/medicare-fee-for-service-payment/snfpps/pdpm">https://www.cms.gov/medicare/medicare-fee-for-service-payment/snfpps/pdpm).

The importance of identifying and treating malnutrition has additional implications. Malnutrition due to undernutrition or overnutrition is recognized as a risk factor for skin integrity issues in vulnerable patients/residents.[11–13]

DISCUSSION
Nutrients, Skin Health, and Wound Healing

Sufficient nutrition is required for skin health and is essential for skin and tissue regeneration. Older adults commonly experience dwindling nutritional status, as evidenced by insidious weight loss, insufficient dietary intake, loss of muscle mass, quality, and strength, declining functional status, and other physical and emotional decline indicators.[14] Undernutrition and its sequelae emerge as an older adult's nutritional well-being diminishes and the elderly become more vulnerable to skin health issues.

Table 1 Coding on minimum data set is associated with increased nontherapy ancillary costs for skilled nursing facility residents	
Description	**Code**
Malnutrition	I5600
Morbid obesity	I8000
Nutritional approaches while a resident, that is, tube feeding or parenteral feeding	K0510A2, K0710A2, K0710B2
Swallowing disorder	K0100A-D
Mechanically altered diet	K0510C2

From Minimum Data Set (MDS) 3.0 Resident Assessment Instrument (RAI) Manual. https://www.cms.gov/medicare/quality/nursing-home-improvement/resident-assessment-instrument-manual.

Sustained pressure, acute trauma, and inflammatory-driven chronic conditions increase the risk for skin integrity issues.[12]

Macronutrients and micronutrients work synergically to maintain skin health and support tissue regeneration. However, aging, disease, and medications often lead to higher nutrient requirements due to impaired nutrient utilization, increased nutrient losses, and increased nutrient needs to restore injured tissues. Energy and protein are the core macronutrients required for each phase of wound healing. When energy intakes are insufficient, the body will utilize carbohydrate and fat stores for energy to support the maintenance and repair of the skin. However, the body does not store excess protein for later use. Protein consists of 20 amino acids of which 9 are indispensable. Protein requirements are based on sufficient intakes of indispensable amino acids (IAA) and nitrogen required for the synthesis of dispensable amino acids and other nitrogen-containing body components.

The body maintains and repairs tissues by utilizing dietary protein and recycled protein from skeletal muscle mass and other organs, that is, liver, kidney, skin, and intestines. Several studies indicate that between 250 to 350 gm of protein is processed each day in healthy adults.[15–17] When dietary intake of IAA from high-quality protein is insufficient to meet needs, that is, wound healing, acute and chronic conditions, and so forth, the body compensates by increasing the breakdown of body proteins resulting in loss of skeletal muscle mass and organ tissues. Moreover, when energy intake is insufficient, protein requirements are increased to meet energy needs and to maintain a positive nitrogen balance.[18,19] Replenishing all protein from organ tissue reserves is essential to maintain total body protein. Failure to do so has cumulative consequences on the overall health and well-being of older adults.[18,20]

In addition to macronutrients, many micronutrients are required to maintain healthy skin. Physical signs of micronutrient deficiencies are often overlooked and laboratory testing to confirm deficiencies is not ordered due to cost. Yet more micronutrient deficiencies are being reported in individuals with obesity,[21] malabsorptive disorders,[21] inflammatory conditions that impair nutrient utilization, self-imposed restrictive diets, food intolerances or allergies, chronic alcohol intakes, and chronic use of medications that interfere with nutrient absorption or promote increased losses.[22–26]

The bulk of research on nutrient requirements for wound healing is specific to pressure injuries; however, the same nutrients support the healing of all intentional and unintentional wounds. **Table 2** summarizes the role of key nutrients to promote skin health and support wound healing. **Table 3** summarizes evidence-based recommendations for macronutrients and oral nutritional supplements (ONS). **Table 4** summarizes evidence-based recommendations for the assessment of micronutrient deficiencies.

Disease-related malnutrition concurrent with pressure injuries and disease-related wounds requires an interprofessional team to prioritize interventions for the medical management of polymorbidities and nutrition interventions. More research is needed on specific nutrients required for individuals with other types of wounds and the impact of pre-existing micronutrient deficiencies on skin health and wound healing.

Cumulative Impact of Malnutrition, Frailty, and Sarcopenia

It is common to see older adults with co-existing undernutrition or malnutrition, frailty, sarcopenia, and inflammatory conditions. With aging, the balance between muscle protein synthesis and muscle protein breakdown dramatically shifts toward more muscle protein breakdown resulting in reduced muscle mass, muscle function deficits, and diminished strength.[27] The overlap of these conditions increases the risk of pressure injuries, chronic wounds, and other geriatric syndromes.[27,28] Moreover,

Table 2
Role of nutrients and recommendations

Nutrients	Role of Key Nutrients
Energy	• Energy, measured in calories, provides fuel for all body functions. • Essential to preserve muscle mass. • Essential to prevent weight loss. • Required for each phase of wound healing.
Protein	• Essential for routine maintenance of the body. • Works synergistically with key nutrients to support collagen synthesis and tissue regeneration. • Required for each phase of wound healing. • Activates microphages and cytokine release during inflammatory phase. • Required for each phase of wound healing.
Carbohydrates	• Provide energy, fiber, flavonoids, and phytonutrients. • Support cell growth, angiogenesis, proliferation of fibroblasts, and leukocytes. • Required for each phase of wound healing.
Hydration (water/beverages)	• Essential for nutrient delivery to wound site, removal of waste products, and tissue perfusion. • Required for each phase of wound healing.
Ascorbic acid	• Essential for the synthesis of neutrophils and collagen. • Activates leukocytes and macrophages. • Involved in collagen cross-linking that gives skin tensile strength. • Required for each phase of wound healing.
B-complex vitamins	• Essential for energy metabolism • Required for inflammation and proliferation phases of wound healing.
Vitamin B12 & Folate	• Involved in erythrocyte maintenance needed for oxygen transport and carbon dioxide removal. • Required for proliferation phase of wound healing.
Vitamin A (beta-carotene and retinol)	• Promotes cell-mediated immune function, collagen synthesis, cross-linking, protein synthesis, and cellular differentiation. • In wounded skin, vitamin A stimulates epidermal turnover, increases the rate of re-epithelialization, and assists the restoration of epithelial structure. • Retinoids enhance the production of the extracellular matrix components, support angiogenesis, and increase proliferation of fibroblasts, keratinocytes. • Required for proliferation and maturation phases of wound healing.
Vitamin E	• Involved in collagen synthesis and cell membrane stabilization. • Required for proliferation phase of wound healing.
Vitamin K	• Essential for blood clotting. • Required for hemostasis phase of wound healing.
Iron	• Involved in collagen synthesis. • Involved in oxygen transport to cells and carbon dioxide removal from cells. • Required for proliferation phase of wound healing.
Zinc	• Involved in protein synthesis, deoxyribonucleic acid synthesis, and cellular growth. • Required for proliferation and maturation phases of wound healing.
Copper	• Involved in collagen cross-linking that gives skin tensile strength. • Component of hemoglobin and is essential for erythrocyte formation. • Required for proliferation and maturation phases of wound healing.

Table 3
Evidence-based recommendations for macronutrients and oral nutritional supplements

Nutrients	Recommendations & Good Practice Statements (GPS) International Guideline, 2019	Other Evidence-Based Guidelines ESPEN Guideline on Nutritional Support for Polymorbid Internal Medicine Patients ESPEN Guidelines for Micronutrient Deficiencies PROT-AGE ESPEN Guidelines for Clinical Nutrition and Hydration in Geriatrics	Implementation Considerations
Energy	4.4: Optimize energy intake for individuals at risk of pressure injuries who are malnourished or at risk of malnutrition. Strength of evidence = B2; Strength of recommendation = ↑ 4.6: Provide 30–35 kcal/kg body weight/d body weight for adults with a pressure injury who are malnourished or at risk of malnutrition Strength of evidence = B2 Strength of recommendation = ↑	R1: The guiding value for energy intake in older persons is 30 kcal/kg body weight/d; this value should be individually adjusted with regard to nutritional status, physical activity level, disease status, and tolerance. Grade B Strong consensus 97% agreement	• Determine energy needs for individuals at risk of or with malnutrition using indirect calorimetry, if available. • Adjust energy intake based on weight change, degree of obesity, and client's medical diagnoses. • Individuals with low BMI may require more energy. • Individuals with BMI of 30 or more need to be evaluated for appropriate intake to promote wound healing. • Dietary restrictions should be modified when limitations result in decreased intake.
Protein Amino acid therapy	4.5: Adjust protein intake for individuals at risk of pressure injuries who are malnourished or at risk of malnutrition. (GPS) 4.7: Provide 1.25–1.5 g/kg body weight/d for adults with a pressure injury who are malnourished or at risk of malnutrition. Strength of evidence = B1 Strength of recommendation = ↑↑	R 2: Protein intake in older persons should be at least 1g protein/kg body weight/d.The amount should be individually adjusted with regard to nutritional status, physical activity level, disease status, and tolerance. Grade B Strong consensus 100% agreement R 5.1: Polymorbid medical inpatients requiring nutritional support shall receive a minimum of 1.0 g of protein/kg of body weight per day in order to prevent body weight loss, reduce the risk of	• High-quality protein provides enough of all indispensable amino acids to achieve positive nitrogen balance. • Protein needs can be met with animal and plant sources of dietary protein. • Assess renal function in context of higher nitrogen load. • Conditionally indispensable amino acids, that may support wound healing in the proliferation phase when total protein and energy needs are met include arginine and citrulline.

(continued on next page)

Table 3
(continued)

Nutrients	Recommendations & Good Practice Statements (GPS) International Guideline, 2019	Other Evidence-Based Guidelines — ESPEN Guideline on Nutritional Support for Polymorbid Internal Medicine Patients; ESPEN Guidelines for Micronutrient Deficiencies PROT-AGE; ESPEN Guidelines for Clinical Nutrition and Hydration in Geriatrics	Implementation Considerations
		complications and hospital readmission, and improve functional outcomes. Grade A strong consensus 95% agreement R 7.1: In polymorbid medical inpatients with pressure ulcers, specific amino-acids (arginine and glutamine) and β-hydroxy-β-methylbutyrate) can be added to oral/enteral feeds to accelerate the healing of pressure ulcers. Grade 0 consensus 90% agreement	• Hydroxymethylbutyrate is a metabolite of leucine that may preserve skeletal muscle mass during inflammatory stress and promote wound healing.
Carbohydrates	No recommendation or good practice statement specific to range of carbohydrate intake.	No recommendation or good practice statement specific to range of carbohydrate intake.	• Quality carbohydrates include unprocessed or minimally processed whole grains, vegetables, fruits, beans. • For clients with dysglycemia, individualize the distribution of carbohydrates and protein during the day to achieve target glucose goals.
Hydration Water/beverages	4.13: Provide and encourage adequate water intake for hydration for an individual with or at risk of a pressure injury, when compatible with goals of care and clinical condition. (GPS)	R 61: Older women should be offered at least 1.6 L of drinks each day, while older men should be offered at least 2.0 L of drinks each day unless there is a clinical condition that requires a different approach. Grade B strong consensus 96% agreement	• Individuals at risk of or with pressure injuries or chronic wounds, provide 30–35 mL/kg body weight of water/beverages per day unless contraindicated or inconsistent with the client's goals. • Up to 20% of water needs may be met from foods. • Provide additional hydration for clients with dehydration, pyrexia, vomiting, diarrhea, hyperhidrosis, and hypernatremia.

Oral Nutritional Supplements Enteral formula	4.10: Provide high-calorie, high-protein, arginine, zinc, and antioxidant oral nutritional supplements or enteral formula for adults with a category/stage 2 or greater pressure injury who are malnourished or at risk for malnutrition Strength of evidence = B1 Strength of recommendation = ↑ 4.11: Discuss the benefits and harms of enteral or parenteral feeding to support overall health in light of preferences and goals of care with individuals at risk of pressure injury who cannot meet their nutritional requirements through oral intake despite nutritional intervention (GPS) 4.12: Discuss the benefits and harms of enteral or parenteral feeding to support pressure injury treatment in light of preferences and goals of care for individuals with pressure injury who cannot meet their nutritional requirements through oral intake despite nutritional interventions Strength of evidence = B1 Strength of recommendation = ↑	R 2.2: In malnourished polymorbid medical inpatients or those at high risk of malnutrition, nutrient-specific ONS should be administered, when they may maintain muscle mass, reduce mortality, or improve quality of life. Grade B strong consensus 89% agreement R 9.3: In polymorbid medical inpatients at high risk of malnutrition or with established malnutrition aged 65 and older, continued nutritional support after hospital discharge with either oral nutritional supplements or individualized nutritional intervention shall be considered to lower mortality. Grade A strong consensus 95% agreement R 52: Nutritional interventions should be offered to older patients at risk of pressure ulcers in order to prevent the development of pressure ulcers. Grade B strong consensus 100% R 53: Nutritional interventions should be offered to malnourished older patients with pressure ulcers to improve healing. Grade B strong consensus 100%	• If oral intake is inadequate, enteral or parenteral nutrition may be recommended if consistent with the individual's wishes. • Enteral (tube) feeding is the preferred route if the gastrointestinal tract is functioning. • Evaluate tolerance to enteral feeding daily.

Abbreviations: BMI, body mass index; ESPEN, European Society for Clinical Nutrition and Metabolism.
Data from Refs.[67–71]

Table 4
Evidence-based recommendations for micronutrients

Nutrients	Recommendations & Good Practice Statements (GPS) International Guideline, 2019 (EPUAP, 2019)	Other Evidence-Based Guidelines ESPEN Guideline on Nutritional Support for Polymorbid Internal Medicine Patients ESPEN Guidelines for Micronutrient Deficiencies PROT-AGE ESPEN Guidelines for Clinical Nutrition and Hydration in Geriatrics GPP	Implementation Considerations
Ascorbic acid	Individualized assessment of ascorbic acid status is required if deficiency is suspected. When physical signs of scurvy are observed and/or laboratory test results confirm deficiency, supplement with ascorbic acid.	R 23.1: Plasma vitamin C concentrations may be measured in all patients with clinical suspicion of scurvy or chronic low intake. Grade of recommendation GPP Consensus 86.84%	• Ascorbic acid is an antioxidant and may decrease inflammation. • Ascorbic acid supports immune response and promotes iron absorption.
B-complex Vitamins	Individualized assessment of thiamine, riboflavin, and niacin status is required if deficiency is suspected. Poor diet, vomiting, and diarrhea contribute to depletion of B-complex vitamin stores. Chronic alcohol intake impairs absorption of thiamine.	R 14.1: Red blood cells or whole blood thiamine may be determined in. • Patients suspected of deficiency in the context of cardiomyopathy and prolonged diuretic treatment. • Patients undergoing a nutritional assessment in the context of prolonged medical nutrition, and post-bariatric surgery. • Refeeding syndrome • Encephalopathy Grade of recommendation 0 Consensus 90% R 15.1: Assessment of riboflavin status can be required when there is clinical suspicion of deficiency. Grade of recommendation GPP Strong consensus 96%	• Many foods are fortified with B-complex vitamins and deficiencies of riboflavin and niacin are uncommon. Untreated thiamine deficiency results in peripheral nerve damage, muscle wasting, myocardial damage.

		R 16.1: In case of clinical symptoms, including diarrhea, dermatitis, and dementia (Pellagra disease), blood or tissue nicotinamide adenine dinucleotide levels may be measured. Grade of recommendation GPP Consensus 89%	
Vitamin B12 & Folate	Individualized assessment of B12 and folate status is required if anemia is suspected. If physical signs of B12 and/or folate deficiency anemia are observed and/or laboratory test results confirm B12 and/or folate deficiency, supplement with B12 and/or folate.	R 20.1: In patients with macrocytic anemia or at risk of malnutrition, folic acid status should be measured at least once at first assessment and repeated within 3 months after supplementation to verify normalization. Grade of recommendation GPP Strong consensus 97% R 20.3: Folate status shall be assessed in plasma or serum (short-term status), or RBC (long-term status) using a method validated against the microbiological assay. Grade of recommendation A Strong consensus 96%	• High intakes of folate may ask a vitamin B12 deficiency.
Vitamin A (beta-carotene and retinol)	Individualized assessment of vitamin A status is required if deficiency is suspected. When physical signs of hypovitaminosis A are observed and/or laboratory test results confirm deficiency, supplement with vitamin A.	R 22.2: Vitamin A status shall be determined by measuring serum retinol. Grade of recommendation A Strong consensus 95%	• Beta-carotene is an antioxidant and may decrease inflammation.
Vitamin E	Individualized assessment of vitamin E status is required if deficiency is suspected. When physical signs of hypovitaminosis E are observed and/or laboratory test results confirm deficiency, supplement with vitamin E.	R 25.1: Vitamin E should be determined when there is clinical suspicion of Vitamin E deficiency. These would include cystic fibrosis, a-beta lipoproteinemia, and thrombotic thrombocytopenic. purpura. In the	• Vitamin E deficiency is rare. • Vitamin E is an antioxidant and may decrease inflammation.

(continued on next page)

Table 4
(continued)

Nutrients	Recommendations & Good Practice Statements (GPS) International Guideline, 2019 (EPUAP, 2019)	Other Evidence-Based Guidelines ESPEN Guideline on Nutritional Support for Polymorbid Internal Medicine Patients ESPEN Guidelines for Micronutrient Deficiencies PROT-AGE ESPEN Guidelines for Clinical Nutrition and Hydration in Geriatrics GPP	Implementation Considerations
		absence of clinical signs of deficiency, there is no indication to measure vitamin E status during parenteral nutrition. Grade of recommendation B Consensus 89%	
Vitamin K	Individualized assessment of vitamin K status is required if deficiency is suspected. When physical signs of hypovitaminosis K are observed and/or laboratory test results confirm deficiency, supplement with vitamin K.	R26.1: The vitamin K status may be measured in at risk patients, including pathologies causing steatorrhea, prolonged use of broad-spectrum antibiotics, and chronic kidney disease. Grade of recommendation GPP Consensus 89%	• Vitamin K deficiency is rare.
Iron	Individualized assessment of iron status is required if anemia is suspected. If physical signs of iron deficiency anemia or anemia of chronic disease are observed and/or laboratory test results confirm etiology of nutritional deficiency, supplement appropriately.	R 9.1: Full investigation of iron status shall be performed in case of anemia, and in case of persistent major fatigue. Grade of recommendation A Strong consensus 94%	• Iron deficiency and anemia of chronic disease are common in older adults due to low-iron diets, chronic use of medications that raise the pH of the stomach, chronic gastrointestinal diseases, and chronic inflammatory disorders.

Zinc	Individualized assessment of zinc status is required if deficiency is suspected. When physical signs of zinc deficiency are observed and/or laboratory test results confirm zinc deficiency, supplement with zinc.	R13.1: Zinc measurement should be done: • In patients with increased gastrointestinal and/or skin losses • On commencing long-term parenteral nutrition, and repeated as required depending on the presence of conditions associated with risk of deficiency. • In patients on long-term parenteral nutrition, every 6–12 months Grade of recommendation GPP Consensus 88%	• Chronic use of 40 mg/d or more supplemental zinc is associated with a copper deficiency and may impair iron absorption as well. Zinc, iron, and copper compete for the same receptor sites in the gut.
Copper	Individualized assessment of copper status is required if deficiency is suspected. When physical signs of copper deficiency are observed and/or laboratory test results confirm copper deficiency, supplement with copper.	R6.1: Copper levels should be measured: • In patients coming for post-bariatric surgery follow-up or • After other abdominal surgeries that exclude the duodenum. • In patients admitted for neuropathy of unclear etiology. • In major burn patients whether receiving complements of copper. • In the context of continuous renal replacement for more than 2 wk. • In patients on home enteral nutrition fed by jejunostomy tubes. • In patients on long term parenteral nutrition, regularly every 6–12 months. Grade of recommendation B Strong consensus 94%	• Copper deficiency is rare. Copper absorption may be impaired in adults taking supplemental zinc more than 40 mg/d.

Abbreviations: BMI, body mass index; ESPEN, European Society for Clinical Nutrition and Metabolism; GPP, good practice point. Data from Refs.[67-71]

the quality of skeletal muscle is negatively impacted by ectopic fat infiltration and is associated with an increased risk for insulin resistance.[29] Preserving muscle mass and optimizing nutrition status are essential for skin health. When skin integrity is breached, the body has fewer resources to support wound healing and regeneration of support tissues.

There is evidence from several randomized controlled trials that demonstrate the role of multi-nutrient ONSs, beta-hydroxy beta-methylbutyrate, vitamin D, and omega-3-fatty acids in reducing the risk for sarcopenia and recovery from surgery when nutrition intake is insufficient.[30–33] Preserving muscle mass and optimizing nutrition status are essential for skin health. When skin integrity is breached the body has fewer resources to support wound healing and regeneration of support tissues.

Other consequences of sarcopenia include sarcopenic obesity and sarcopenic dysphagia.[27,34–37] Older adults with obesity often have decreased muscle mass and decreased strength due to aging. However, the progressive loss of muscle quality is primarily due to fatty infiltration in muscles. Individuals with sarcopenic obesity are at greater risk of poor health-related outcomes than either obesity or sarcopenia alone.[38] Diagnostic criteria for sarcopenic obesity proposed by the European Society for Clinical Nutrition and Metabolism (ESPEN) and the European Association for the Study of Obesity expert panels include assessment for low muscle mass and impaired muscle function concurrent with excess adiposity. Sarcopenic obesity is further stratified by the presence of clinical complications associated with obesity and dysfunction of skeletal muscle.[39]

Oropharyngeal dysphagia is associated with a higher risk of malnutrition and pressure injuries in older adults.[40] While the most common etiologies of dysphagia are due to neurologic causes, Japanese professional organizations focused on dysphagia, sarcopenia, and rehabilitation nutrition have published an evidence-based diagnostic algorithm for sarcopenic dysphagia. The diagnostic algorithm for sarcopenic dysphagia excludes neurologic etiologies of dysphagia (Fujishima, 2019).[34] Sarcopenic dysphagia has been reported in individuals with dysphagia caused by sarcopenia of the swallowing muscles.[35–37] Characteristics of older adults identified with sarcopenic dysphagia include prolonged nil per os or nothing by mouth orders, unnecessary inactivity, and insufficient nutritional intake. More research is needed to examine the role of nutrition in the prevention and treatment of sarcopenic dysphagia.

Nutrition Care Guideline

The Academy of Nutrition and Dietetics has established a systematic method that nutrition professionals use to provide nutrition care. The nutrition care process (NCP), consists of a 4-step process of assessment, nutrition diagnosis, nutrition interventions, and monitoring/evaluation.[41] Application of the NCP, along with interprofessional team collaboration, and the implementation of individualized nutrition interventions have been linked to improved nutritional clinical outcomes in individuals at risk for or with actual malnutrition.[42]

Nutritional screening

Few things are as essential as ensuring that individuals receiving health care have adequate nutritional status. Poor nutritional status can have an impact on both wound development and wound healing.[12] A nutrition screening can be performed in any practice. Nutrition screening tools should be appropriate for the population being evaluated, valid, and reliable. Examples of valid and reliable nutrition screening tools that are sensitive indicators of risk for developing wounds include the Mini Nutritional Assessment and the Malnutrition Universal Screening Tool.[28,43]

While the nutrition screening parameters are defined by the registered dietitian/nutritionist (RDN), the screening process should be carried out by other members of the health care team who have been deemed competent in the use of the screening tool.[44] Any member of the interprofessional team can be trained to conduct a nutritional screening. Individuals identified at nutritional risk should be referred to the RDN for an in-depth nutrition assessment to be conducted.

As outlined in the 2019 International Guideline nutrition recommendations, a nutritional screening should be conducted on all individuals identified as at risk for developing pressure injuries.[12] See **Table 5** for a list of validated nutrition screening tools.[45–57]

Nutrition assessment

The completion of a nutrition assessment involves the evaluation of data collected through conducting a food and nutrition-related history, evaluating biochemical data, looking at anthropometric measurements, conducting a nutrition-focused physical examination, reviewing medical tests and procedures, appraising the ability to eat independently, and utilizing evidence-based guidelines to compare all data collected.[12,58] Research supports that the use of an interprofessional nutrition protocol in individuals with stage 2 and 3 pressure injuries can result in improved wound healing.[59]

Laboratory studies such as serum albumin, prealbumin, and other laboratory values may be useful in establishing the overall prognosis for the patient but are not considered sensitive indicators of nutritional status. Research reveals that changes in acute-phase proteins do not reliably or predictably change with weight loss, calorie restriction, or nitrogen balance.[12] Serum protein levels can be affected by inflammation, renal function, hydration, and other factors. Inflammatory biomarkers are not recommended for the diagnosis of malnutrition.[12,60] These markers seem to reveal the severity of inflammatory response rather than nutritional status. The presence of inflammation augments the risk of malnutrition by altering the body's metabolism and influencing protein utilization. This renders the relevance of laboratory values as indicators of malnutrition limited.[12]

Anthropometric measurements offer direct or indirect information about body composition. These measurements are suitable for evaluating an individual's nutritional status as well as monitoring the outcomes of nutrition interventions.[58]

A comprehensive physical examination is a vital element of the nutrition assessment. A nutrition-focused examination begins with a general overview of appearance, height, weight, growth, ascites, and edema. RDNs aim to identify loss of muscle or fat mass, decreased functional status, poor oral intake, and increased body weight due to inflammation-related fluid accumulation. A nutrition-focused physical assessment is essential in identifying single multiple nutrient deficiencies to define appropriate and timely treatment.

Nutrition Interventions and Wound Healing

Basic nutrition care for individuals with wounds relies on food-first tactics. Providing individuals with their favorite foods and encouraging and promoting adequate intake are key to promoting improvement in nutritional status. Approaches to boost adequate intake involve providing nutrition counseling, offering fortified foods, liberalizing dietary restrictions, helping with meals, respecting cultural and ethnic preferences, and providing a pleasant dining environment (to name a few).

Individuals with chronic diseases might be hypermetabolic when the body is inefficient in processing the nutrients consumed. The use of ONS can be an effective intervention to help meet the kilocalorie and protein needs of individuals at risk for

Table 5
Summary of the nutrition screening tool validation studies

Nutrition Screening Tool	Evidence for Identifying Pressure Injury Risk Status	Evidence for Identifying Factors Associated with Pressure Injury Risk	Clinical Setting
Mini Nutritional Assessment full version (MNA®)[45]	Yes	Yes	Older adults in community settings[28]
			Older adults in long-term care[46]
			Older adults with pressure injuries and multiple comorbidities[47]
			Older adults at nutritional risk in long-term care and community settings[48]
			Older adults in acute care, long-term care, and community settings[49]
Malnutrition Universal Screening Tool (MUST)[50]	No	Yes	Older adults in acute care, long-term care, and community settings[49]
Nutrition Risk Screening (NRS) 2002[51]	No	No	Adults in acute care[52]
			Older adults in acute care, long-term care, and community settings[49]
Short Nutrition Assessment Questionnaire (SNAQ)[53,54]	No	No	Adults in acute care[55]
			Older adults in residential care[55]
Seniors in the Community: Risk Evaluation for Eating and Nutrition (SCREEN©)[56,57]	No	No	Older adults in community settings[56]

With permission from European Pressure Ulcer Advisory Panel, National Pressure Injury Advisory Panel and Pan Pacific Pressure Injury Alliance. Prevention and Treatment of Pressure Ulcers/Injuries: Clinical Practice Guideline. The International Guideline. Emily Haesler (Ed.). EPUAP/NPIAP/PPPIA; 2019.

developing wounds, that cannot meet their needs through a standard (regular) diet. The 2019 International clinical practice guideline provides support for the use of ONS with micronutrients for individuals with a wound who are malnourished (or at risk) (see **Table 3**). Research supports that using ONS can result in positive energy balance and clinical benefits, especially if ONS (1.5–2.4 kcal/mL) is consumed between meals.[12]

Individualized Care Plan

For individuals with, or at risk of developing, wounds who are malnourished or who are at risk of malnutrition, outlining an individualized care plan and communicating the plan's goals and interventions with the care providers is the last step of the nutrition assessment.

When developing a nutrition care plan, care should be taken to ensure that the plan is customized for everyone. The individual's wishes and preferences, along with inputs from the interprofessional team, should guide the process. Smart goals with a review schedule and a completion date, followed by specific interventions that the patient has agreed to should be added to the medical record. Changes in medical conditions, positive and negative, call for care plan revisions.

Impact of Chronic Disease on Nutrition and Wound Healing

The nutrition care of individuals with wounds goes much further than the skin injury. In most instances, comorbidities that are managed through medical nutrition therapy must be attended to in an effort to impact wound care. The presence of chronic diseases, such as diabetes mellitus (DM) and impaired glucose tolerance (prediabetes), heart failure, atrial fibrillation (Afib), chronic obstructive pulmonary disease (COPD), renal insufficiency, anemia, and dementia can contribute to malnutrition and serve as a risk factor for wound development.

Uncontrolled blood glucose levels can also inhibit wound healing. Uncontrolled hyperglycemia causes the cell walls to become stiff and rigid, decreasing the blood flow through the small vessels present on the wound surface. Uncontrolled DM can contribute to reduced oxygen being released from the hemoglobin molecule thus decreasing the availability of oxygen and nutrients in the wound site.[61]

Oxygen is vital for all stages of wound healing. Conditions that are linked with low tissue oxygen tension might upsurge the risk of developing wounds. Conditions such as heart failure, Afib, myocardial infarction, and COPD fall under this category.[61]

Individuals with chronic kidney disease or end-stage renal disease on hemodialysis treatment, often develop a uremic state that creates metabolic disturbances affecting many organ systems, including the gastrointestinal tract. The decrease in motility can contribute to anorexia and overall reduced intake of food and fluids.[62]

Confusion and agitation are observed in individuals suffering from dementia. As changes in cognition progress, individuals will need assistance with meals, have decreased sensations of hunger and thirst, or do not recognize foods at all. This can contribute to an increased risk of malnutrition and reduced healing rate.[63]

Nutrition Care at End of Life

Immobility, serious illness, and poor prognosis place patients at risk for developing wounds during the end stages of life. Individualized interventions should be implemented after the benefits and harm of the therapy have been thoroughly discussed with the patient, family, and/or caregivers. The Academy of Nutrition and Dietetics and ESPEN support that individuals have the right to request or refuse nutrition and hydration as a medical treatment after adequate information (education) has been provided.[64,65]

While the intake of food and fluids is generally considered indispensable to maintaining life and supporting healing, in some cases, the sustained delivery of food and fluids can no longer benefit a patient and may cause harm. At the end of life, patients have decreased caloric needs. Providing nutrients and fluids based on previously calculated nutritional needs can lead to edema, heart failure, and pulmonary congestion.[66] At the end of life, patients normally do not experience hunger or thirst. Decreased intake and weight loss is a normal development of end-of-life disease.[64,65] The lack of food and fluid promotes ketosis in the body and releases opioids in the brain, which may create a sense of euphoria.[64,65] Provisions should be made for individuals who wish to consume food and fluids at the end stage of life.

CLINICS CARE POINTS

Consuming a healthy diet and sufficient fluids is crucial to promote wound healing. Nutrients are needed in the right amount and combination to stimulate tissue growth and regeneration. No individual nutrient stands alone as the sole substrate to replenish devitalized tissue with healthy tissue. In the following section are a few care points to incorporate into your practice.

- Conduct a nutrition screening to identify actual malnutrition or risk for malnutrition in every patient.

- Individuals screened at risk of malnutrition or who are malnourished should be referred to the RDN to complete an in-depth nutrition assessment.

- Individuals with a wound or at risk of developing wounds should be referred to the RDN so that an in-depth nutrition assessment can be conducted.

- The interprofessional team should collaborate to develop an individualized plan of care.

- Patients should be encouraged to consume a healthy diet that meets their nutritional needs.

- ONS should be provided to all individuals who cannot meet their nutritional needs with a standard (regular diet alone).

DISCLOSURE

The authors have nothing to disclose.

REFERENCES

1. Pappas A, Liakou A, Zouboulis CC. Nutrition and skin. Rev Endocr Metab Disord 2016;17(3):443–8.
2. Cao C, Xiao Z, Wu Y, et al. Diet and skin aging-from the perspective of food nutrition. Nutrients 2020;12(3):870.
3. Visioli F, Marangoni F, Poli A, et al. Nutrition and health or nutrients and health? Int J Food Sci Nutr 2022;73(2):141–8.
4. Perez FP, Perez CA, Chumbiauca MN. Insights into the social determinants of health in older adults. J Biomed Sci Eng 2022;15(11):261–8.
5. Cardenas D, Correia MITD, Hardy G, et al. The international declaration on the human right to nutritional care: a global commitment to recognize nutritional care as a human right. Clin Nutr 2023;42(6):909–18.
6. Tobert CM, Mott SL, Nepple KG. Malnutrition diagnosis during adult inpatient hospitalizations: analysis of a multi-institutional collaborative database of academic medical centers. J Acad Nutr Diet 2018;118(1):125–31.

7. Smith LO, Vest MT, Rovner AJ, et al. Prevalence and characteristics of starvation-related malnutrition in a mid-Atlantic healthcare system: a cohort study. J Parenter Enteral Nutr 2022;46(2):357–66.
8. World Health Organization. Malnutrition. World Health Organization; 2021. Available at: https://wwwwhoint/news-room/q-a-detail/malnutrition. Accessed 15 July, 2023.
9. Center for Disease Control and Prevention. Provisional Mortality Statistics. 2018 through Last Month Request (June 7, 2023). 2023. Accessed 15 July, 2023. http://wonder.cdc.gov/mcd-icd10-provisional.html.
10. Moloney L, Jarrett B. Nutrition assessment and interventions for the prevention and treatment of malnutrition in older adults: an evidence analysis center scoping review. J Acad Nutr Diet 2021;121(10):2108–40.
11. AoNa Dietetics. Malnutrition in older adults. Evidence Analysis Library; 2023. https://www.andeal.org/topic.cfm?menu=6064. Accessed 15 July, 2023.
12. *European pressure ulcer advisory Panel, national pressure injury advisory Panel and Pan pacific pressure injury alliance. Prevention and Treatment of pressure ulcers/injuries: clinical practice guideline.* European pressure ulcer advisory Panel, national pressure injury advisory Panel and Pan pacific pressure injury alliance. In: Haesler E, editor. EPUAP/NPIAP/PPPIA. The international guideline. 2019.
13. Munoz N, Litchford MD, Cox J, et al. Malnutrition and pressure injury risk in vulnerable populations: application of 2019 international clinical practice guideline. Adv Skin Wound Care 2022;35(3):136–65.
14. Behavioral CBO, Adults L in O. Social Isolation and Loneliness in Older Adults. 2020. Available at: https://www.shareable.net/wp-content/uploads/2019/07/Shareable_community-solutions-to-the-loneliness-epidemic.pdf.
15. Medicine Io. Dietary Reference Intake National Academy Press. 2005. Accessed 15 July, 2023. https://nap.nationalacademies.org/read/10490/chapter/1.
16. Reeds PJ, Garlick PJ. Nutrition and protein turnover in man. Advanced Nutrition Research 1984;6:93–138.
17. Waterlow JC. Protein turnover with special reference to man. Q J Exp Physiol 1984;69:409–38.
18. Pasini E, Corsetti G, Aquilani R, et al. Protein-amino acid metabolism disarrangements: the hidden enemy of chronic age-related conditions. Nutrients 2018;10(4):391.
19. Pellett PL. Protein-energy interactions. Lausanne, Switzerland: Scrimshaw eds IDECG; 1992. p. 81–121.
20. Nishimura Y, Musa I, Holm L, et al. Recent advances in measuring and understanding the regulation of exercise-mediated protein degradation in skeletal muscle. American Journal of Physiology-cell Physiology 2021;321(2):C276–87.
21. Parrott J, Frank LL, Rabena R, et al. American society for metabolic and bariatric surgery integrated health nutritional guidelines for the surgical weight loss patient 2016 update: micronutrients. Surg Obes Relat Dis 2017;13(5):727–41.
22. Ceppa EP, Valsangkar N, Schmidt H, et al. Is Scurvy a 21st century diagnosis? implications on surgical patients. Ann Clin Nutr 2019;2(1):1013.
23. Esper D. Utilization of nutrition-focused physical assessment in identifying micronutrient deficiencies. Nutr Clin Pract 2015;30(2):194–202.
24. Filippi J, Al-Jaouni R, Wiroth JB, et al. Nutritional deficiencies in patients with Crohn's disease in remission. Inflamm Bowel Dis 2006;12(3):185–91.
25. Harries AD, Heatle R. Nutritional disturbances in Crohn's disease. Postgrad Med 1983;59(697):690–7.

26. Vidarsdottir JB, Johannsdottir SE, Thorsdottir I, et al. A cross-sectional study on nutrient intake and -status in inflammatory bowel disease patients. Nutr J 2016; 15(1):61.

27. Rasheedy D, EL-Kawaly WH. The cumulative impact of sarcopenia, frailty, malnutrition, and cachexia on other geriatric syndromes in hospitalized elderly. Electronic Journal of General Medicine 2021;18(2):em277.

28. Grattagliano I, Marasciulo L, Paci C, et al. The assessment of the nutritional status predicts the long term risk of major events in older individuals. Eur Geriatr Med 2017;8(3):273–4.

29. Correa-de-Araujo R, Addison O, Miljkovic I, et al. Myosteatosis in the context of skeletal muscle function deficit: an interdisciplinary workshop at the national institute on aging. Front Physiol 2020;11:963.

30. Deutz NE, Matheson EM, Matarese LE, et al. Readmission and mortality in malnourished, older, hospitalized adults treated with a specialized oral nutritional supplement: a randomized clinical trial. Clin Nutr 2016;35(1):18–26.

31. Ekinci O, Yanık S, Terzioğlu Bebitoğlu B, et al. Effect of calcium β-Hydroxy-β-methylbutyrate (CaHMB), Vitamin D, and protein supplementation on postoperative immobilization in malnourished older adult patients with hip fracture: a randomized controlled study. Nutr Clin Pract 2016;31(6):829–35.

32. Malafarina V, Uriz-Otano F, Malafarina C, et al. Effectiveness of nutritional supplementation on sarcopenia and recovery in hip fracture patients. A multi-centre randomized trial. Maturitas 2017;101:42–50.

33. Matheson EM, Nelson JL, Baggs GE, et al. Specialized oral nutritional supplement (ONS) improves handgrip strength in hospitalized, malnourished older patients with cardiovascular and pulmonary disease: a randomized clinical trial. Clin Nutr 2021;40(3):844–9.

34. Fujishima I, Fujiu-Kurachi M, Arai H, et al. Sarcopenia and dysphagia: position paper by four professional organizations. Geriatr Gerontol Int 2019;19(2):91–7.

35. Maeda K, Takaki M, Akagi J. Decreased skeletal muscle mass and risk factors of sarcopenic dysphagia: a prospective observational cohort study. J Gerontol A Biol Sci Med Sci 2017;72(9):1290–4.

36. Takagi D, Hirano H, Watanabe Y, et al. Relationship between skeletal muscle mass and swallowing function in patients with Alzheimer's disease. Geriatr Gerontol Int 2017;17(3):402–9.

37. Wakabayashi H, Takahashi R, Watanabe N, et al. Prevalence of skeletal muscle mass loss and its association with swallowing function after cardiovascular surgery. Nutrition 2017;38:70–3.

38. Bouchonville MF, Villareal DT. Sarcopenic obesity: how do we treat it? Curr Opin Endocrinol Diabetes Obes 2013;20(5):412–9.

39. Donini LM, Busetto L, Bischoff SC, et al. Definition and diagnostic criteria for sarcopenic obesity: ESPEN and EASO consensus statement. Obes Facts 2022; 15(3):321–35.

40. Banda KJ, Chu H, Kang XL, et al. Prevalence of dysphagia and risk of pneumonia and mortality in acute stroke patients: a meta-analysis. BMC Geriatr 2022; 22(1):420.

41. Posthauer ME, Banks M, Dorner B, et al. The role of nutrition for pressure ulcer management: national pressure ulcer advisory panel, european pressure ulcer advisory panel, and pan pacific pressure injury alliance white paper. Adv Skin Wound Care 2015;8:175–88.

42. Sriram K, Sulo S, VanDerBosch G, et al. A comprehensive nutrition-focused quality improvement program reduces 30-day readmissions and length of stay in hospitalized patients. JPEN - J Parenter Enter Nutr 2017;41:384–91.

43. Tsaousi G, Stavrou G, Ioannidis A, et al. Pressure ulcers and malnutrition: results from a snapshot sampling in a University Hospital. Med Princ Pract 2015; 24(1):11–6.

44. Academy of Nutrition and Dietetics. Evidence Analysis Library Web Site. 2018. Accessed 24 July, 2023. https://www.andeal.org/topic.cfm?menu=5382.

45. Nestle Nutrition Institute. Mini Nutritional Assessment MNA®. Nestlé. May 2019. https://www.mna-elderly.com/forms/mini/mna_mini_english.pdf.

46. Langkamp-Henken B, Hudgens J, Stechmiller JK, et al. Mini nutritional assessment and screening scores are associated with nutritional indicators in elderly people with pressure ulcers. J Am Diet Assoc 2005;105(10):1590–6.

47. Hengstermann S, Fischer A, Steinhagen-Thiessen E, et al. Nutrition status and pressure ulcer: what we need for nutrition screening. JPEN - J Parenter Enter Nutr 2007;31(4):288.

48. Tsai AC, TL C, YC W, et al. Population-specific short-form mini nutritional assessment with body mass index or calf circumference can predict risk of malnutrition in community-living or institutionalized a people in Taiwan. J Am Diet Assoc 2010; 110(9):1328–34.

49. Poulia KA, Yannakoulia M, Karageorgou D, et al. Evaluation of the efficacy of six nutritional screening tools to predict malnutrition in the elderly. Clin Nutr 2012; 31(3):378–85.

50. BAPEN. Malnutrition Universal Screening Tool. May 2019. https://www.bapen.org.uk/pdfs/must/must-full.pdf.

51. Kondrup J, Allison SP, Elia M, et al, Educational and Clinical Practice Committee, European Society of Parenteral and Enteral Nutrition ESPEN. ESPEN guidelines for nutrition screening 2002. Clin Nutr 2003;22(4):415–21.

52. Kondrup J, Rasmussen HH, Hamberg I, et al. Nutritional risk screening (NRS 2002): a new method based on an analysis of controlled clinical trials. Clin Nutr 2003;3:321–36.

53. Dutch Malnutrition Steering Group. SNAQ English. Dutch malnutrition steering group 2019. https://www.fightmalnutrition.eu/?s=SNAQ+English.

54. Dutch Malnutrition Steering Group. SNAQ (various languages). Dutch Malnutrition Steering Group; 2019. https://www.fightmalnutrition.eu/?s=SNAQ.

55. Neelemant F, Kruizenga HM, de Vet HC, et al. Screening malnutrition in hospital outpatients. Can the SNAQ malnutrition-screening tool also be applied to this population? Clin Nutr 2008;27(3):439–46.

56. Keller HH, Goy R, Kane SL. Validity and reliability of SCREEN II (Seniors in the Community: risk evaluation for eating and nutrition, version II). Eur J Clin Nutr 2005;59:1149–57.

57. Flintbox. SCREEN©. Seniors in the community risk evaluation for eating and nutrition. Wellspring Worldwide, LLC; 2019. https://www.flintbox.com/public/project/2750.

58. Academy of Nutrition and Dietetics. Nutrition care manual. Academy of Nutrition and Dietetics; 2023. http://www.nutritioncaremanual.org/. Accessed 7/25/2023.

59. Allen B. Effects of a comprehensive nutritional program on pressure ulcer healing, length of hospital stay, and charges to patients. Clin Nurs Res 2013;22(2):186–205.

60. White J, Guenter P, Jensen G, et al. Consensus Statement: AND and ASPEN: characteristics recommended for the identification and documentation of adult malnutrition (undernutrition). J Acad Nutr Diet 2012;112(5):730–8.

61. Guo S, DiPietro LA. Factors affecting wounf healing. J Dent Res 2010;89(3): 219–29. https://www.ncbi.nlm.nih.gov/pmc/articles/PMC2903966/. Accessed 7/26/21.

62. Maroz N, Simman R. Wound healing in patients with impaired kidney function. J Am Coll Clin Wound Spec 2014;5(1):2–7.

63. Jaul E, Meiron O. Dementia and pressure ulcers: is there a close pathophysiological interrelation? J Alzheimers Dis 2017;56(3):861–6.

64. Druml C, Ballmer PE, Druml W, et al. ESPEN guideline on ethical aspects of artificial nutrition and hydration. Clin Nutr 2016;35(3):545–56.

65. O'Sullivan-Maillet J, Schwartz DB, Posthauer ME, et al. Ethical and legal issues in feeding and hydration. J Acad Nutr Diet 2013;113(6):828–33.

66. Groher ME, Groher TP. When safe oral feeding is threatened: end-of-life options and decisions. Top Lang Disord 2012;32(2):149–67.

67. Haesler E ed. European Pressure Ulcer Advisory Panel, National Pressure Injury Advisory Panel, and Pan Pacific Pressure Injury Alliance. 2019.

68. Gomes F, Schuetz P, Bounoure L, et al. ESPEN guidelines on nutritional support for polymorbid internal medicine patients. Clin Nutr 2018;37(1):336–53.

69. Berger MM, Shenkin A, Schweinlin A, et al. ESPEN micronutrient guideline. Clin Nutr 2022;41(6):1357–424.

70. Bauer J, Biolo G, Cederholm T, et al. Evidence-based recommendations for optimal dietary protein intake in older people: a position paper from the PROT-AGE Study Group. J Am Med Dir Assoc 2013;14(8):542–59.

71. Volkert D, Beck AM, Cederholm T, et al. ESPEN guideline on clinical nutrition and hydration in geriatrics. Clin Nutr 2019;38(1):10–47.

The Chronic Wound–Related Pain Model

Holistic Assessment and Person-Centered Treatment

Kevin Woo, PhD, RN, NSWOC, WOCC(C)

KEYWORDS

- Chronic wounds • Wound pain model • Wound related pain

KEY POINTS

- Chronic wound related pain may vary based on wound etiologies and treatment related factors.
- Atraumatic dressing may mitigate chronic wound related pain that is often caused by tissue trauma at wound dressing changes.
- Increased pain is one of the signs associated with wound infection that warrants careful evaluation and prompt treatment.
- Pain assessment should be part of routine wound care during rest and wound dressing change.
- Topical or systemic pharmacotherapy for the treatment of pain is determined by pain types (nociceptive versus neuropathic), symptom pattern (intensity, onset, duration), characteristics of the medication (available routes of administration, dosing intervals, side effects) and individual factors (eg, age, coexisting diseases).

INTRODUCTION

Wound healing involves complex sequential processes that require a delicate interplay and balance of different cells, extracellular matrix, cytokines, and growth factors for the restoration of skin integrity.[1] Deviation or defects from the normal healing trajectory lead to chronic wounds that may last for years and exhibit signs of protracted and excessive inflammatory responses. These difficult-to-heal wounds are estimated to affect 1.67 per 1000 people globally at any given time and will continue to increase due to a rapidly aging population and growing incidence of obesity, diabetes, and vascular diseases.[2] The exorbitant societal and economic toll on the health system and individuals for ongoing care and management is well documented and indisputable. With growing

Faculty of Health Sciences, Queen's University, 92 Barrie Street, Kingston, Ontario K7L 3N6, Canada
E-mail address: Kevin.woo@queensu.ca

Clin Geriatr Med 40 (2024) 501–514
https://doi.org/10.1016/j.cger.2023.12.013   **geriatric.theclinics.com**

awareness and prioritization of patient safety and quality improvement in wound care, patient-reported outcome measures are gaining ground. In a recent systematic review of reported experiences in the treatment of complex wounds, Raepsaet and colleagues[3] identified 82 possible outcomes that were clustered into 5 categories, including pain and comfort as a primary concern in receiving wound care. While wound healing is a desirable outcome, our attention should turn to wound-related pain, which is ubiquitous and the most disabling symptom that intrudes into every aspect of a person's life. This article will describe the multidimensionality of chronic wound–related pain and appraise the evidence on management strategies.

To capture the inherent subjectivity and diversity of pain experiences, the International Association for the Study of Pain redefined pain as "an unpleasant sensory and emotional experience associated with, or resembling that is associated with, actual or potential tissue damage."[4] This definition eloquently speaks to the many faces of pain that can categorized into (1) nociceptive pain caused by actual or threatened tissue damage from a specific noxious stimulus (eg, inflammation or ischemia), (2) neuropathic pain that arises from disturbances of somatosensory nervous system, and (3) nociplastic pain caused by persistent inflammation. Chronic wound–related pain is often underassessed and undertreated. In a recently systematic review pooling data from 10 studies, the investigators reported that 80% of persons living with venous leg ulcers (VLUs) experience mild-to-moderate pain at rest in between dressing changes.[5] Tegene and colleagues[6] examined pain in 424 hospitalized patients with a variety of acute and chronic wounds; all study participants expressed mild-to-severe pain during wound management. Regrettably, most patients (94%) received no pain treatment. Suboptimal management of pain may stem from the lack of awareness and knowledge deficit. According to a survey of 512 nurses in Italy,[7] over 87% of the respondents acknowledged that they did not possess adequate knowledge to conduct pain assessments on their patients with wounds and 81% did not understand how to document pain. These results raise questions about routine wound care practices that may contribute to pain and the lack of knowledge in assessing and managing pain.

Based on the biopsychosocial approach to examining pain, the chronic wound–related pain model posits that pain can be triggered by wound-related or treatment-related factors and modulated by our thinking, emotions, social context, environment, and personal factors (**Fig 1**).[8–10] The aim is to help guide comprehensive pain assessment and management strategies for people living with chronic wound–related pain.

Wound Types and Pain

A pressure injury (PI) refers to localized cutaneous damage as a consequence of excessive or prolonged pressure or shear to the skin and contiguous underlying tissue. The combined results of ischemia-reperfusion injury, lymphatic channel obstruction, cellular deformation contribute to elevated inflammation, reactive oxygen species production, and apoptosis or cell death.[11] Inflammatory mediators engender complex changes in peripheral and central signal processing by activating the nociceptors, evoking pain or modulating the sensitivity of the primary nociceptors. In fact, pain is an early sign that heralds pressure injuries.[12]

Diabetic foot ulcers are among the most common and insidious complications for people living with diabetes mellitus that can lead to severe infection and amputation. Depending on geographic locations, the documented prevalence of painful diabetic peripheral neuropathy ranges from 10% to 70%.[13] Neuropathic pain is usually spontaneous and manifests itself in a wide range of presentations from allodynia (pain evoked by a stimulus that does not normally provoke pain), dysesthesia, hyperalgesia

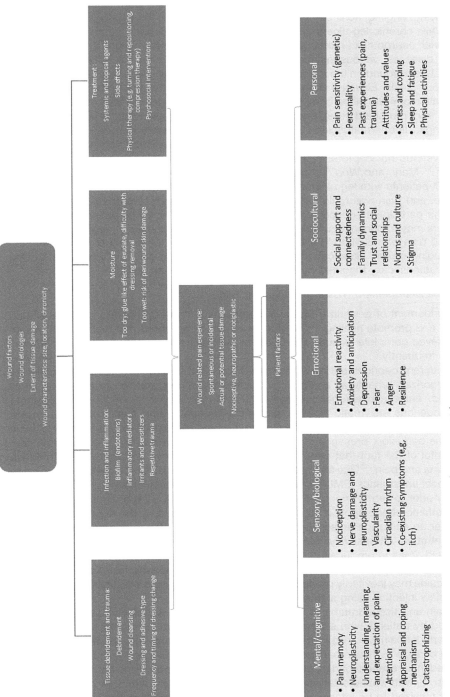

Fig. 1. Chronic wound–related pain. (*Courtesy of K. Woo 2023.*)

(intensified pain from a noxious stimulus) to paresthesia (anomalous sensations of prickling, tingling, itching).[13,14]

While chronic leg ulcers may involve an array of underlying pathologies including arterial, neuropathic, metabolic, hematological, infectious, malignant, and inflammatory diseases, venous insufficiency predominantly accounts for 70% of all cases.[15] A VLU is a wound on the lower leg caused by an underlying vascular disease involving venous stasis. Elevated venous pressure promotes extravasation and dermal accumulation of white blood cells, growth factors, fibrin, and hemosiderin (ferritin and ferric iron from red blood cells), precipitating painful conditions including eczematous skin changes, lipodermatosclerosis, edema, vasculopathy, and eventually ulcerations.[15,16] Localized release of proinflammatory cytokines and mediators activates venous and perivenous nociceptors, resulting in excruciating throbbing, burning, and stinging pain.[17] Marin and Woo[18] conducted a retrospective analysis of data collected from 1007 patients with leg ulcers; 263 (26%) of participants had evidence of arterial disease, and pain was ranked as one of the most common symptoms with two-thirds of the participants describing pain as moderate/severe. While patients with arterial ulcers may experience a wide range of clinical symptoms, the predominant concern is leg pain with 82% to 100% of patients experiencing persistent or temporary pain including classic claudication and cramping pain in the calves, thighs, or buttocks, characteristically triggered by exertion and subsiding with rest.[19]

Tissue Debridement, Tissue Trauma, and Pain

Debridement of devitalized tissue is a necessary step to prepare an optimal wound bed and promote healing.[20,21] Nearly twice as many venous and diabetic foot ulcers achieved complete closure with frequent debridement compared with those treated less frequently.[21]

Different debridement methods have been used in clinical practice, and they are categorized broadly as sharp/surgical, mechanical (eg, wet to dry dressing), ultrasonic, enzymatic (exogenous enzymes), autolytic (moist wound bed to promote endogenous enzymatic activity), biological (maggots), and oxidative.[20] The choice of debridement method is contingent on the type and extent of tissue damage, local tissue perfusion, presence of infection, available resources, and patient preference; mindful of the fact that certain methods are nonselective and more likely to cause trauma and pain.[22] Oral analgesics or local anesthetic such as topical eutectic mixture of local anesthetics (EMLA) cream should be offered to patients and timed appropriately prior to debridement.[23] Proper application of EMLA is important to optimize local anesthetic effect: apply a thick layer of the topical agent on the exposed tissue and under an occlusion dressing or plastic wrap for 30 to 60 minutes to enhance tissue penetration. Alternatively, lidocaine 1% solution (10 mg/cc) can be injected into periwound areas to produce fast (within seconds) analgesic effect. This drug is relatively safe but should be limited to 3 mg/kg of lidocaine. Upon local injection into the skin, lidocaine may inevitably produce an intense burning sensation that can be ameliorated by slow injection using a small-gauge needle.[24]

Pain and tissue trauma at wound dressing changes is well established. As elucidated by patients who suffered from painful chronic wounds in their interviews, the severity of pain was largely determined by how the wound was handled during dressing change by health care professionals.[25] Using a repeated measure design, Woo asked their research participants to rate their pain before dressing change, at dressing removal, with wound cleansing, and after dressing reapplication.[26] Although pain was hypothesized to be intensified during change, the finding that pain scores were the highest during wound cleansing was surprising. It is possible that derangements in pain sensitization have rendered individuals hypersensitive to light touch and pressure that is otherwise innocuous. Meticulous wound hygiene is part of an important step to remove debris, foreign material, dead cells, and excess drainage.[27] Gentle rinsing is inadequate but more aggressive techniques such as using an abrasive woven gauze to wipe over the wound surface can potentially be damaging. Striking the balance is at the core of the issue. Rajhathy and her research team sought to examine the evidence on whether wound cleansing using either irrigation or swabbing techniques have an impact on pain, bleeding, infection, and characteristics of wound tissue.[28] Only 1 study was eligible for the review and they concluded that wound swabbing was associated with increased pain and increased rates of infection as opposed to irrigation. Routine wound cleansing should incorporate the following best practice recommendations to lessen discomfort.[29]

- Avoid excessive irrigation pressure (4–15 PSI is recommended).
- Choose cleansing agents with surfactant to helping separation and removal of tenacious devitalized tissue.
- Irrigate wounds with an adequate volume of solution (50–100 mL/cm of wound length).
- Warm cleansing solution to appropriate temperature (room temperature or slightly warmer).
- Cleanse the peri-wound skin to remove exudate, effluent, debris, scale and/or to control skin flora.
- Avoid concentrated and cytotoxic antiseptics that may cause stinging and pain.
- Apply saline or antiseptic-soaked gauze compress and allow it dwell on wound surface for 5 to 10 minutes.

Dressings removal can also be unpleasant. Depending on the dressing material and adhesives, pulling of the dressing away from the fragile skin and detaching wound tissue along with congealed exudate that is embedded in the dressing microstructure can be damaging to the wound and excruciatingly painful to patients. If excessive peel force is required, there is an appreciable risk for skin stripping and medical adhesive–related skin injury (MARSI), as evident by persistent erythema and blisters, and skin tears.[30] This is especially true for negative pressure wound therapy (NPWT), which promotes tissue ingrowth into specialized porous foam dressing. Bleeding from removing foam dressing that is firmly attached to wound surface is a common occurrence.[31] Placing an interface between the foam and wound surface, inactivating therapy 15 to 30 minutes before scheduled dressing change, and administering fluid in the NPWT tubing into the sponge are strategies to reduce traumatic dressing removal and pain.[31]

With the advent of innovative material and technologies, a plethora of modern dressings are available. The prudent selection of dressings with an atraumatic wound contact layer, like silicone, has been documented to limit skin damage/trauma with dressing removal and to minimize pain at dressing changes.[32] Silicones are inert synthetic polymers that pose no toxicity risk; they are arranged in long chains of siloxanes cross-linked with molecules like carbon, hydrogen, and oxygen. Silicones are known for temperature stability, compressibility, and resistance to shear stress and weathering; these advantages lend credence to widespread interest in using silicone for other medical devices and personal care products such as implants (breasts and penis), insulating pacemaker and cardioverter-defibrillator leads, sports equipment, and housewares. As wound care products, soft silicone dressings are coated with a hydrophobic soft silicone contact layer that yields ideal wettability and low surface tension to maintain a moist wound environment without damaging the fragile tissue.[33,34] Once attached to the skin, the silicone layer forms a stable and immediate seal between the wound-dressing interface to minimize lateral fluid movement and aid fluid absorption vertically into the absorbent core. In comparison to other adhesives, the silicone coatings do not become more adhesive during dressing wear time, yet they allow the dressing to be reapplied multiple times without loss of adhesion and apply less mechanical strain on skin during removals than other dressing types. In light of their unique properties and adequate performance in biomechanical testing of peel forces, silicone dressings are widely popular in wound care, PI prevention and treatment of radiation dermatitis, and scar management.[34,35]

Waring and colleagues[36] compared 6 different modern wound dressings and their potential for skin stripping and impairment of the skin's barrier function. Stratum corneum was found on all dressings except a soft silicone foam dressing. Similarly, Matsumura and colleagues[37] demonstrated that wound dressings coated with a silicone adhesive incurred significantly less detachment of the stratum corneum and regenerating epithelium, followed by other dressings coated with polyurethane, hydrocolloid, and acrylic adhesives. Leblanc and Woo[38] completed a randomized controlled trial (RCT) to examine the effectiveness of soft silicone atraumatic dressing versus nonadherent dressings on the management of skin tears. Participants who were randomized to receive soft silicone dressings required less frequent changes and achieved faster healing by 50% compared with those randomized to nonadherent/non-silicone dressings. By limiting unnecessary dressing changes, natural wounds healing is allowed without interruption, unnecessary exposure to cold ambient air, and increased risk of contamination. The International Skin Tear Advisory Panel advocates the use of nonadherent/silicone tapes or foam dressings for skin tear management to avoid stripping or tearing of the skin.[39] To minimize pain at dressing change and MARSI, consider removing dressings slowly, taking small areas at a time, aiming at a low angle of traction, applying counter-traction (with an index finger) and using adhesive solvents when necessary. All in all, silicone dressing may facilitate undisturbed wound healing and promote cost-effectiveness to achieve desirable clinical outcomes.

Wound-related pain may be referred to areas that are extended beyond the wound margins and more pronounced in the surrounding periwound skin. When the volume of drainage exceeds the fluid-handling capacity of the dressing material, enzyme-rich and caustic exudate may spill over to wound margins, causing maceration, tissue erosion, and pain. Maceration of the periwound skin typically presents as white, wrinkled, soggy tissue at the wound edge.[39] In a crossover RCT, patients with wound margin maceration and skin damage were found to experience increased pain even before dressing changes.[40] Putative solutions may include using absorbent dressing materials such as gelling fiber, alginate, foams, and superabsorbent polymer–containing wound dressings. Skin barriers, sealants, and protectants with zinc, petrolatum, acrylate, and cyanoacrylate are available in wipes, sprays, gels, and liquid roll-ons to use prophylactically for protecting fragile skin.[41] By preventing maceration and tissue damage, these products are designed to reduce wound-related pain and improve the overall healing process.

Sudden emergence or exacerbation of wound-related pain has been well validated as one of the clinical indicators for increased bioburden, therefore warrants careful evaluation.[42] Recent advances in the understanding of wound infection have generated tremendous interest in biofilm, a complex community of microbial cells that is enclosed firmly in an extracellular polysaccharide substance.[43] Biofilms release toxins, bacterial deoxyribonucleic acid fragments, matrix proteins, and other molecules, and they play a key role in perpetuating inflammatory cellular response and cutaneous innate immune response, invoking noticeable but subtle changes in wounds including inflamed granulation tissue (granulitis), excessive drainage, odor, and pain.[44]

There is insufficient evidence to substantiate the routine use of systemic antimicrobials to catalyze wound healing. In fact, concerted efforts are being put in place to promote judicious antibiotic prescribing to curb resistance. Early detection to guide prompt treatment of local infection with topical antimicrobial agents may be more effective in preventing pathogens from invading into deeper tissue compartment and causing more serious infections. Various dressings with silver, polyhexamethylene biguanide,[45] cadexomer iodine,[46] gentian violet/methylene blue,[47] and honey[48] have been used successfully to manage infection with a significant improvement in pain as one of the surrogate markers or diagnostic criteria. These topical antimicrobials are relatively safe with minimal side effects, systemic absorption, and resistance reported in the literature. No one dressing is more superior. If healing becomes stalled after a minimum of 2-week challenge, clinicians may consider replacing the existing treatment with an entirely different type of antimicrobials.[29] To achieve better outcomes, antimicrobial dressings should be used in conjunction with serial and ongoing debridement to mechanically disrupt and combat biofilm.[29]

THE MULTIDIMENSIONS OF CHRONIC WOUND–RELATED PAIN

While wound pain has been linked to elevated biomarkers such as interleukin (IL)-1β and IL-6, the pain experience cannot be solely inferred from excessive inflammations and biological aberrations.[49] Pain is highly subjective and personal. A vast array of mental/cognitive, emotional, sensory/biological, social, and personal factors are interwoven together like skeins to form the tapestry of pain experiences that differ considerably across individuals. This complexity means substantial heterogeneity exists in the presentations of pain and responses to treatments. Of the 13 potential predictors of pain during dressing changes, expected or anticipatory pain intensity prior to dressing change was categorically the most powerful predictor of pain during dressing change; the more pain expected, the more severe pain experienced at dressing change.[50] Anticipation or negative expectation of impending pain has been demonstrated to activate certain neurocircuitry that facilitates pain transmission, a phenomenon also known as nocebo hyperalgesia.[26] In a study of 96 patients with chronic wounds, Woo[26] reported that patients who experienced high levels of anxiety also reported high levels of anticipatory pain, leading to high levels of pain at dressing change. The result is a vicious cycle of pain, stress/anxiety, and worsening of pain. Similar relationship between anxiety and wound-related pain has been validated in studies of patients with burn wounds,[51] VLUs, and ischemic leg wounds.[52] Building a therapeutic relationship through mutual and collaborative approaches is central to allay anxiety, align expectations, and establish realistic expectations. To establish trust and cultivate a therapeutic alliance, clinicians must first acknowledge that anxiety and pain are common experiences at dressing changes. While patients should be informed that these symptoms are part of a normal response, emphasis should be placed on available treatment options and achievable goals to minimize them. Pain-related education is a necessary step to debunk common misconceptions and myths that may obstruct effective pain management. Patients are respected for their roles to be active participants who make informed choices for their wound treatment. By placing patient in the center of care, the intentionality of self-management is to augment patients' skills and confidence in managing their wounds, monitoring progress, setting realistic treatment goals, and problem-solving.[53] Patients may find self-management appealing because they can find the most suitable time for wound treatment with minimal disruption to their lifestyle. Patients reported less pain, more empowered, and better quality of life.[53]

Consequences of Chronic Wound–Related Pain

No matter how fleeting it may appear, recurrent experiences of pain during dressing changes can have a lasting effect. Based on results from previous studies, pain is a potent stressor that triggers a cascade of neuroendocrine response precipitating elevated levels of stress hormones such as cortisol, catecholamines, and vasopressin.[10,54] These physiologic changes not only heighten pain sensitivity but also impede wound healing by compromising normal metabolic functions, inflammatory response, local circulation, and immune defense mechanisms. In a meta-analysis of 17 studies, Walburn and colleagues[55] validated the significant relationship between stress and wound healing; the higher the level of stress, the slower the healing process. Clinicians should be cognizant of how pain can threaten patients' ability and willingness to adhere to care activities that are central to the prevention and improvement of PU/PI: turning and repositioning, changing soiled clothing, following a recommended skin care regime, and taking adequate nutrition. While limiting physical activity is a natural strategy to avoid exertional pain, pain-related fear of movement may lead to greater disability affecting social engagement and participation in meaningful activities.[56,57] People with venous disease require life-long maintenance compression therapy to attenuate vein distension and edema. Over half of the patients with VLUs were unable to tolerate compression therapy because of wound pain.[58] Poor adherence to compression may contribute to the recurrence rate of VLUs; estimating 26% after 1 year of complete closure.[58,59] In addition to pain, adherence to compression therapy could be a challenge in the older population due to reduced dexterity, muscle strength, range of motion, and flexibility.[59] Potentials solutions may include assistive devices and lower levels of compression. Pentoxifylline, flavonoids, (such as Escin, hydroxyethylrutoside, and Daflon), zinc, and anti-inflammatory drugs that promote healing of VLUs may also have the potential to attenuate pain.[60] Holistic, comprehensive assessment should encompass the impact of pain on low energy level, fatigue, limitations in activities, lost work productivity, depression, sleep disturbance, pervasive stigma, and social isolation.

Pharmacotherapy for Chronic Wound–Related Pain

Pharmacotherapy is the mainstay treatment which may vary based on the type (nociceptive vs neuropathic), pain pattern (intensity, onset, duration), characteristics of the medication (available routes of administration, dosing intervals, side effects), and individual factors (eg, age, coexisting diseases, and other over-the-counter or herbal medications).[61,62] Whether the pain is of nociceptive or neuropathic origin, selection of appropriate pharmaceuticals should always take into account the characteristics of the drug (eg, onset, duration, available routes of administration, dosing intervals, side effects) and individual factors (eg, age, coexisting diseases, and other over-the-counter or herbal medications).

Nonopioid pharmacologic therapies such as acetaminophen, nonsteroidal anti-inflammatory drugs (NSAIDs), selected antidepressants, and anticonvulsants are preferred for chronic pain management. Opioids are not recommended for first-line or routine therapy for subacute or chronic pain, and they can be addictive, misused, abused, and diverted.[61] Realizing the risk of short-term opioid use can lead to unintended long-term opioid use, opioid should always be started at the lowest effective dose; a daily dosage of 20 to 30 MME/day for opioid-naïve patients at the beginning until reaching recommended dosages of 50 to 90 MME/day, a threshold beyond which pain improvement is less noticeable.[61] Clinically meaningful improvement is defined as a 30% improvement in pain, function, and/or quality of life.[61] Opioids should then be tapered as pain resolves and discontinued as soon as feasible.

Neuropathic pain is refractory to treatment; symptoms may improve with adjuvant treatments such as tricyclic, tetracyclic, and serotonin and norepinephrine reuptake inhibitor antidepressants; selected anticonvulsants (eg, pregabalin, gabapentin enacarbil, oxcarbazepine); and capsaicin and lidocaine patches.[62,63] Duloxetine and pregabalin have been approved for the treatment of diabetic peripheral neuropathy. Unique to patients with open cutaneous wounds, topical application of morphine, tricyclic antidepressants (eg, amitriptyline), NSAIDs, capsaicin, ketamine, lidocaine/prilocaine, and nitroglycerin ointment (for ischemic pain only) have been used with the added advantage of local effect and minimal systemic side effects.[45,64,65] Topical morphine is thought to act on opioid receptors found in the structures including the peripheral nerves, hair follicles, melanocytes, and various cells of the immune system.[64] Burgeoning research interest focuses on the potential use of cannabinoids to help assuage pain in light of their anti-inflammatory and antioxidant properties.[65]

Nonpharmacologic treatments are almost as effective as opioids in pain management. These approaches span from distraction and relaxation techniques such as guided imagery, exercise, massage, cognitive therapy, music, and hypnosis,[66–68] to more technical or digital solutions such as virtual reality, computer games, visual stimulation, and electrical stimulation.[68–72] Evidence also lends credence to the use of support groups that brings people living with wounds together to socialize and share information. The objectives are to reduce the potential effect of psychological contributors to pain (such as anxiety and stress), modify beliefs, build self-efficacy, and foster effective coping. Depending on the type and location of the wound, patients may find therapeutic surfaces, leg elevation, and rest helpful.

Chronic Wound–Related Pain Measurement

Pain assessment should be part of routine wound care during rest and wound dressing change. There is no one instrument that can meet the diverse needs of people living with chronic wound pain, the choice may vary on account of individual's age, developmental stage, cognitive status, communication abilities, and cultural predisposition. Categorical scales, numerical rating scales, pain thermometers, visual analog scales, FACES scales, and verbal categorical scales are easy to use, single-dimensional tools designed for patients to quantify pain intensity, unpleasantness, or extent to which pain relief is experienced.[72] Descriptions of pain quality, such as those incorporated on the McGill Pain Questionnaire, have been validated for the differentiation of nociceptive from neuropathic pain. Uncommon tactile and thermal sensations associated with numbness, tingling, pins and needles, burning, shooting, and electric shocklike sensation are typical features of neuropathic pain that can be measured by the Neuropathic Pain Scale, Neuropathic Pain Symptom Inventory, and the Diabetic Peripheral Neuropathic Pain Impact Measure.[72] Concomitant neurologic examination should consider assessment of motor, sensory, and autonomic involvement to identify all signs of neurologic dysfunction. In general, objective assessment methods are less reliable; they may include physiologic indicators, biomarkers, behaviors or facial expressions, and functional performance. To obtain a comprehensive assessment of pain, multidimensional measurements (eg, Brief Pain Inventory) are available to evaluate the many facets of pain and its impact on daily functioning, mood, social functioning, and other aspects of quality of life.

SUMMARY

Chronic wound–related pain is shaped by biopsychosocial factors. In this article, a conceptual framework is proposed to highlight the vicissitudes of the pain experience. Troublesome pain symptoms may evolve from one or more sources, including wound etiologies and local wound care such as surgical debridement procedures or dressing changes. A multimodal and multidisciplinary approach to a pain management approach to wound care is necessary to address these comorbid conditions and psychosocial issues in addition to selecting appropriate wound care and dressing options. Timely, appropriate, holistic, compassionate, and person-centered care and treatment is key. Proper management of pain during wound care can also help attenuate the physiologic stress response, promote treatment adherence, and improve patient outcomes.

CLINICS CARE POINTS

- Patients living with chronic wounds experience pain that can be described as nociceptive, neuropathic, and nociplastic.
- Atraumatic dressings with silicone reduce injury to periwound skin and granulating wound bed at dressing removal and promote better wound healing.
- Dressings which contain antimicrobial agents including silver, polyhexanide, cadexomer iodine, gentian violet/methylene blue, and honey are effective against local wound infection as evident by significant improvement in pain as one of the surrogate markers.
- Anticipation or negative expectation of impending pain can exacerbate pain experience, a phenomenon also known as nocebo hyperalgesia.
- Nonopioid pharmacologic therapies such as acetaminophen, NSAIDs, selected antidepressants, and anticonvulsants are preferred for chronic pain management.
- Opioids are not recommended for first-line or routine therapy for subacute or chronic pain; the risk of short-term opioid use can lead to unintended long-term opioid use.
- Opioid should always be used at the lowest effective dose and then be tapered as pain resolves and discontinued as soon as feasible.
- Topical application of morphine, tricyclic antidepressants (eg, amitriptyline), NSAIDs, capsaicin, ketamine, lidocaine/prilocaine, and cannabinoids have been used for wound-related pain treatment with the added advantage of local effect and minimal systemic side effects.

DISCLOSURE

The author has nothing to disclose.

REFERENCES

1. Tan MLL, Chin JS, Madden L, et al. Challenges faced in developing an ideal chronic wound model. Expet Opin Drug Discov 2023;18(1):99–114.
2. Martinengo L, Olsson M, Bajpai R, et al. Prevalence of chronic wounds in the general population: systematic review and meta-analysis of observational studies. Ann Epidemiol 2019;29:8–15.
3. Raepsaet C, Alves P, Cullen B, et al. Clinical research on the use of bordered foam dressings in the treatment of complex wounds: a systematic review of

reported outcomes and applied measurement instruments. J Tissue Viability 2022;31(3):514–22.

4. Raja SN, Carr DB, Cohen M, et al. The revised International Association for the Study of Pain definition of pain: concepts, challenges, and compromises. Pain 2020;161(9):1976–82.

5. Leren L, Johansen E, Eide H, et al. Pain in persons with chronic venous leg ulcers: a systematic review and meta-analysis. Int Wound J 2020;17(2):466–84.

6. Tegegne BA, Lema GF, Fentie DY, et al. Severity of wound-related pain and associated factors among patients who underwent wound management at teaching and referral hospital, northwest Ethiopia. J Pain Res 2020;13:2543–51.

7. Toma E, Veneziano ML, Filomeno L, et al. Nursing assessment of wound-related pain: an Italian Learning survey. Adv Skin Wound Care 2020;33(10):540–8.

8. Woo KY, Sibbald RG. Chronic wound pain: a conceptual model. Adv Skin Wound Care 2008;21(4):175–88.

9. Woo KY, Abbott LK, Librach L. Evidence-based approach to manage persistent wound-related pain. Curr Opin Support Palliat Care 2013;7(1):86–94.

10. Woo KY. Exploring the effects of pain and stress on wound healing. Adv Skin Wound Care 2012 Jan;25(1):38–44.

11. Pan Y, Yang D, Zhou M, et al. Advance in topical biomaterials and mechanisms for the intervention of pressure injury. iScience 2023;26(6):106956.

12. Wilson H, Moore Z, Avsar P, et al. Exploring the role of pain as an early indicator for individuals at risk of pressure ulcer development: a systematic review. Worldviews Evidence-Based Nurs 2021;18(4):299–307.

13. Preston FG, Riley DR, Azmi S, et al. Painful diabetic peripheral neuropathy: practical guidance and challenges for clinical management. Diabetes Metab Syndr Obes 2023;16:1595–612.

14. Jang HN, Oh TJ. Pharmacological and nonpharmacological treatments for painful diabetic peripheral neuropathy. Diabetes Metab J 2023;47(6):743–56.

15. Krizanova O, Penesova A, Hokynkova A, et al. Chronic venous insufficiency and venous leg ulcers: aetiology, on the pathophysiology-based treatment. Int Wound J 2023. https://doi.org/10.1111/iwj.14405.

16. Chaudhry S, Lee K. Diagnosing and managing venous stasis disease and leg ulcers. Clin Geriatr Med 2024;40(1):75–90.

17. Guo X, Gao Y, Ye X, et al. Experiences of patients living with venous leg ulcers: a qualitative meta-synthesis. J Tissue Viability 2023;S0965-206X(23):00132–8.

18. Marin JA, Woo KY. Clinical characteristics of mixed arteriovenous leg ulcers: a descriptive study. J Wound, Ostomy Cont Nurs 2017;44(1):41–7.

19. Horváth L, Németh N, Fehér G, et al. Epidemiology of peripheral artery disease: narrative review. Life 2022;12(7):1041.

20. Nowak M, Mehrholz D, Barańska-Rybak W, et al. Wound debridement products and techniques: clinical examples and literature review. Postepy Dermatol Alergol 2022;39(3):479–90.

21. Thomas DC, Tsu CL, Nain RA, et al. The role of debridement in wound bed preparation in chronic wound: a narrative review. Ann Med Surg (Lond) 2021;71:102876.

22. Rajhathy EM, Chaplain V, Hill MC, et al. Executive summary: debridement: Canadian best practice recommendations for nurses developed by nurses specialized in wound, ostomy and continence Canada (NSWOCC). J Wound, Ostomy Cont Nurs 2021;48(6):516–22.

23. Briggs M, Nelson EA, Martyn-St James M. Topical agents or dressings for pain in venous leg ulcers. Cochrane Database Syst Rev 2012;11(11):CD001177.

24. McBride CA, Wong M, Patel B. Systematic literature review of topical local anaesthesia or analgesia to donor site wounds. Burns Trauma 2022;10:tkac020.

25. Probst S, Gschwind G, Murphy L, et al. Patients 'acceptance' of chronic wound-associated pain - a qualitative descriptive study. J Tissue Viability 2023;32(4): 455–9.

26. Woo KY. Unravelling nocebo effect: the mediating effect of anxiety between anticipation and pain at wound dressing change. J Clin Nurs 2015;24(13–14): 1975–84.

27. Murphy C, Atkin L, Vega de Ceniga M, et al. Embedding Wound Hygiene into a proactive wound healing strategy. J Wound Care 2022;31(Sup4a):S1–19.

28. Rajhathy EM, Meer JV, Valenzano T, et al. Wound irrigation versus swabbing technique for cleansing noninfected chronic wounds: a systematic review of differences in bleeding, pain, infection, exudate, and necrotic tissue. J Tissue Viability 2023;32(1):136–43.

29. Swanson T, Ousey K, Haesler E, et al. IWII wound infection in clinical practice consensus document: 2022 update. J Wound Care 2022;31(Sup12):S10–21.

30. Hitchcock J, Haigh DA, Martin N, et al. Preventing medical adhesive-related skin injury (MARSI). Br J Nurs 2021;30(15):S48–56.

31. Apelqvist J, Willy C, Fagerdahl AM, et al. Negative pressure wound therapy – overview, challenges and perspectives. J Wound Care 2017;26(Suppl 3):S1–113.

32. LeBlanc K, Langemo D, Woo K, et al. Skin tears: prevention and management. Br J Community Nurs 2019;24(Sup9):S12–8.

33. Woo K, Kasaboski J. A pilot retrospective study to evaluate two multi-layer foam dressings for the management of moderately exudative pressure injuries. Surg Technol Int 2017;31:61–5.

34. Gefen A, Alves P, Beeckman D, et al. How should clinical wound care and management translate to effective engineering standard testing requirements from foam dressings? mapping the existing gaps and needs. Adv Wound Care 2022. https://doi.org/10.1089/wound.2021.0173.

35. Gefen A, Alves P, Beeckman D, et al. Mechanical and contact characteristics of foam materials within wound dressings: theoretical and practical considerations in treatment. Int Wound J 2022. https://doi.org/10.1111/iwj.14056.

36. Waring M, Bielfeldt S, Mätzold K, et al. An evaluation of the skin stripping of wound dressing adhesives. J Wound Care 2011;20(9):416–22.

37. Matsumura H, Imai R, Ahmatjan N, et al. Removal of adhesive wound dressing and its effects on the stratum corneum of the skin: comparison of eight different adhesive wound dressings. Int Wound J 2014;11(1):50–4.

38. LeBlanc K, Woo K. A pragmatic randomised controlled clinical study to evaluate the use of silicone dressings for the treatment of skin tears. Int Wound J 2022; 19(1):125–34.

39. LeBlanc K, Beeckman D, Campbell K, et al. Best practice recommendations for prevention and management of periwound skin complications. Wounds International; 2021. Available online at: www.woundsinternational.com.

40. Woo KY, Coutts PM, Price P, et al. A randomized crossover investigation of pain at dressing change comparing 2 foam dressings. Adv Skin Wound Care 2009;22(7): 304–10.

41. Dissemond J, Assenheimer B, Gerber V, et al. Moisture-associated skin damage (MASD): a best practice recommendation from Wund-D.A.CH. J Dtsch Dermatol Ges 2021;19(6):815–25.

42. Eriksson E, Liu PY, Schultz GS, et al. Chronic wounds: treatment consensus. Wound Repair Regen 2022;30(2):156–71. Erratum in: Wound Repair Regen. 2022 Jul;30(4):536.
43. Haesler E, Swanson T, Ousey K, et al. Establishing a consensus on wound infection definitions. J Wound Care 2022;31(Sup12):S48–59.
44. Hill R, Woo K. A prospective multisite observational study incorporating bacterial fluorescence information into the UPPER/LOWER wound infection checklists. Wounds 2020;32(11):299–308.
45. Ffrench C, Finn D, Velligna A, et al. Systematic review of topical interventions for the management of pain in chronic wounds. Pain Rep 2023;8(5):e1073. Erratum in: Pain Rep. 2023 Oct 10;8(6):e1105.
46. Woo K, Dowsett C, Costa B, et al. Efficacy of topical cadexomer iodine treatment in chronic wounds: systematic review and meta-analysis of comparative clinical trials. Int Wound J 2021;18(5):586–97.
47. Woo KY, Heil J. A prospective evaluation of methylene blue and gentian violet dressing for management of chronic wounds with local infection. Int Wound J 2017;14(6):1029–35.
48. Holubová A, Chlupáčová L, Krocová J, et al. The use of medical grade honey on infected chronic diabetic foot ulcers-A prospective case-control study. Antibiotics (Basel) 2023;12(9):1364.
49. Goto T, Saligan LN. Wound pain and wound healing biomarkers from wound exudate: a scoping review. J Wound, Ostomy Cont Nurs 2020;47(6):559–68.
50. Gardner SE, Bae J, Ahmed BH, et al. A clinical tool to predict severe pain during wound dressing changes. Pain 2022;163(9):1716–27.
51. Sahin AT, Sahin SY. Influence of burn specific pain anxiety on pain experienced during wound care in adult outpatients with burns. Burns 2023;49(6):1335–43.
52. Kelechi TJ, Muise-Helmericks RC, Theeke LA, et al. An observational study protocol to explore loneliness and systemic inflammation in an older adult population with chronic venous leg ulcers. BMC Geriatr 2021;21(1):118.
53. Kapp S, Santamaria N. The effect of self-treatment of wounds on quality of life: a qualitative study. J Wound Care 2020;29(5):260–8.
54. Stojadinovic O, Gordon KA, Lebrun E, et al. Stress-induced hormones cortisol and epinephrine impair wound epithelization. Adv Wound Care 2012;1(1):29–35.
55. Walburn J, Vedhara K, Hankins M, et al. Psychological stress and wound healing in humans: a systematic review and meta-analysis. J Psychosom Res 2009;67(3):253–71.
56. Klein TM, Andrees V, Kirsten N, et al. Social participation of people with chronic wounds: a systematic review. Int Wound J 2021;18(3):287–311.
57. Qiu Y, Team V, Osadnik CR, et al. Barriers and enablers to physical activity in people with venous leg ulcers: a systematic review of qualitative studies. Int J Nurs Stud 2022;135:104329.
58. Zhang L, Chen J, Ning N, et al. Measuring patient compliance with wearing graduated compression stockings. J Vasc Surg Venous Lymphat Disord 2023;11(1):46–51.e2.
59. Bar L, Brandis S, Marks D. Improving adherence to wearing compression stockings for chronic venous insufficiency and venous leg ulcers: a scoping review. Patient Prefer Adherence 2021;15:2085–102.
60. Kitchens BP, Snyder RJ, Cuffy CA. A literature review of pharmacological agents to improve venous leg ulcer healing. Wounds 2020;32(7):195–207.

61. Dowell D, Ragan KR, Jones CM, et al. CDC clinical practice guideline for prescribing opioids for pain — United States, 2022. MMWR Recomm Rep (Morb Mortal Wkly Rep) 2022;71(No. RR-3):1–95.
62. Clauw DJ, Essex MN, Pitman V, et al. Reframing chronic pain as a disease, not a symptom: rationale and implications for pain management. Postgrad Med 2019; 131(3):185–98.
63. Neuropathic pain in adults: pharmacological management in non-specialist settings. London: National Institute for Health and Care Excellence (NICE); 2020.
64. Patel R, Mogoi RO, Ali SK. Topical lidocaine and morphine gel use for malignant wound pain. J Pain Palliat Care Pharmacother 2023;37(3):216–7.
65. Healy CR, Gethin G, Pandit A, et al. Chronic wound-related pain, wound healing and the therapeutic potential of cannabinoids and endocannabinoid system modulation. Biomed Pharmacother 2023;168:115714.
66. Pombeiro I, Moura J, Pereira MG, et al. Stress-reducing psychological interventions as adjuvant therapies for diabetic chronic wounds. Curr Diabetes Rev 2022;18(3). e060821195361.
67. Chester SJ, Tyack Z, De Young A, et al. Efficacy of hypnosis on pain, wound-healing, anxiety, and stress in children with acute burn injuries: a randomized controlled trial. Pain 2018;159(9):1790–801.
68. Zamani Kiasari A. Effect of foot reflexology massage on pain and pain anxiety severity during dressing change in burn patients. Burns 2022;48(8):2012–3.
69. Zheng L, Liu H. Virtual reality distraction, a novel tool for pain alleviation during dressing change following surgical drainage of perianal abscess at Day Treatment Centre. Digit Health 2023;9. 20552076231155675.
70. Milne J, Swift A, Smith J, et al. Electrical stimulation for pain reduction in hard-to-heal wound healing. J Wound Care 2021;30(7):568–80.
71. He ZH, Yang HM, Dela Rosa RD, et al. The effects of virtual reality technology on reducing pain in wound care: a meta-analysis and systematic review. Int Wound J 2022;19(7):1810–20.
72. Holloway S, Ahmajärvi K, Frescos N, et al. Holistic management of wound-related pain. J Wound Management 2023;23(2 Sup1).

Moving?

Make sure your subscription moves with you!

To notify us of your new address, find your **Clinics Account Number** (located on your mailing label above your name), and contact customer service at:

Email: journalscustomerservice-usa@elsevier.com

800-654-2452 (subscribers in the U.S. & Canada)
314-447-8871 (subscribers outside of the U.S. & Canada)

Fax number: 314-447-8029

**Elsevier Health Sciences Division
Subscription Customer Service
3251 Riverport Lane
Maryland Heights, MO 63043**

*To ensure uninterrupted delivery of your subscription, please notify us at least 4 weeks in advance of move.

9780443246500